Giant-Cell Arteritis

Edited by Imtiaz A. Chaudhry

Published in London, United Kingdom

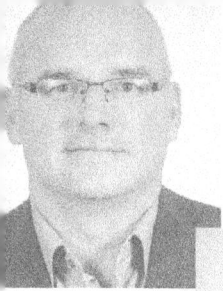
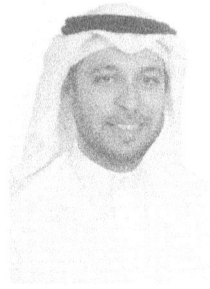
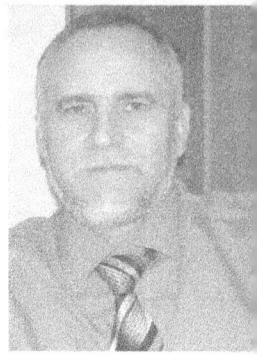
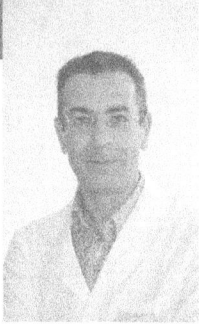
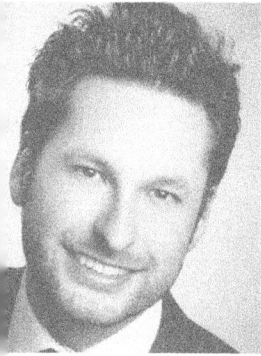
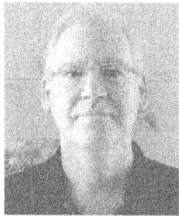
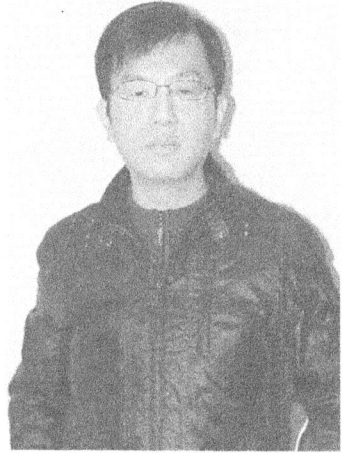

IntechOpen

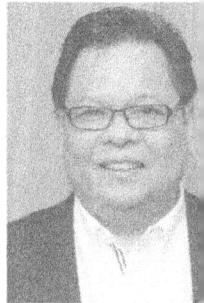
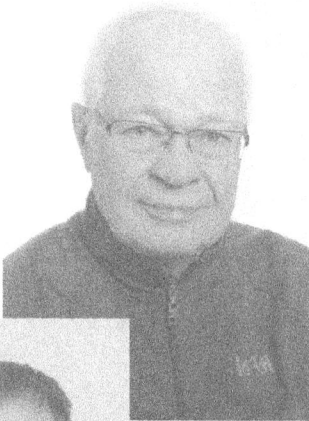
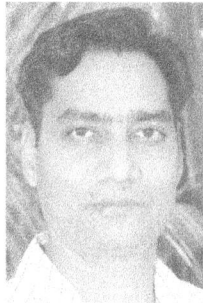
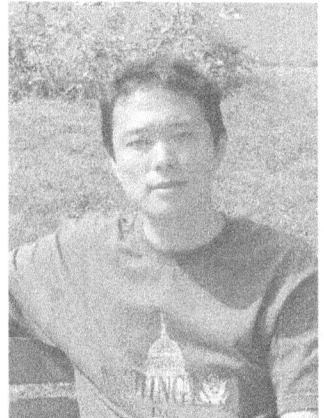
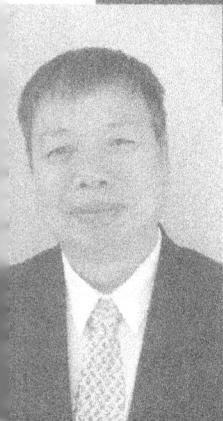
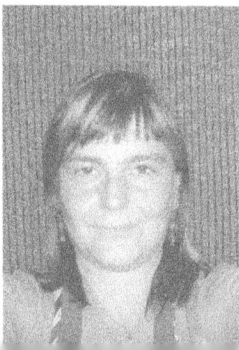

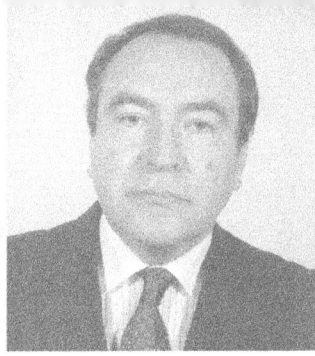

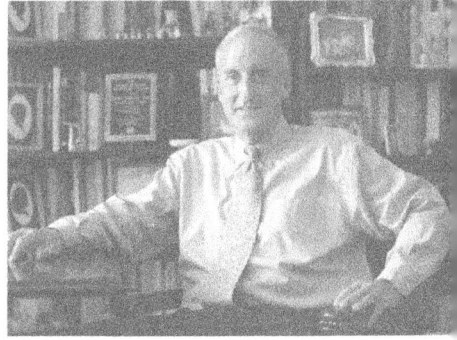

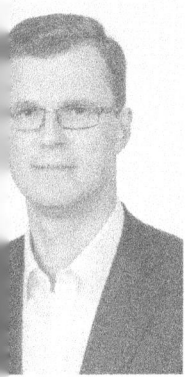

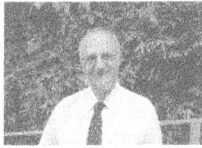

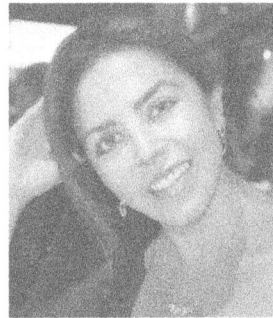

Supporting open minds since 2005

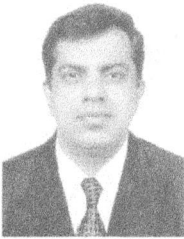

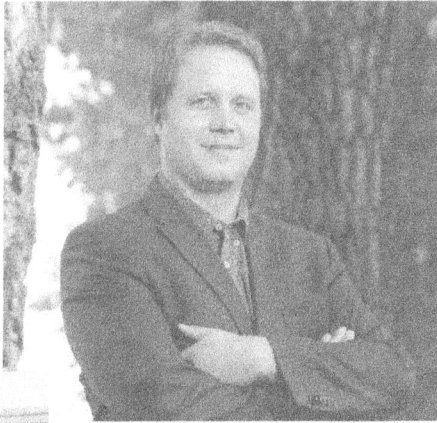

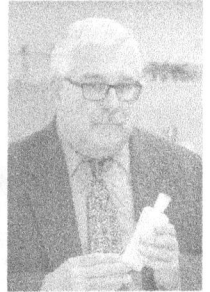

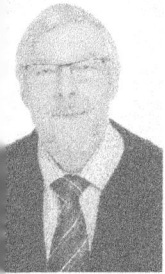

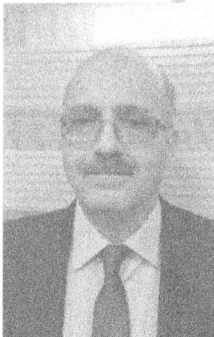

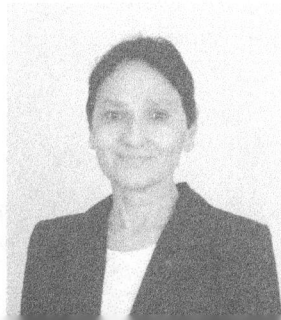

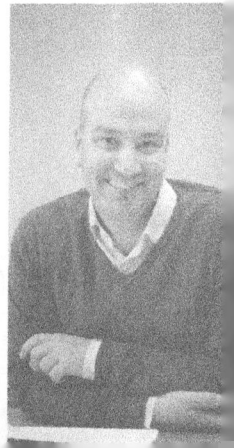

Giant-Cell Arteritis
http://dx.doi.org/10.5772/intechopen.91490
Edited by Imtiaz A. Chaudhry

Contributors
Dragoș Cătălin Jianu, Silviana Nina Jianu, Georgiana Munteanu, Traian Flavius Dan, Ligia Petrica,
Radwan Qasrawi, Diala Abu Al-Halawa, Omar Daraghmeh, Mohammad Hjouj, Rania Abu Sier, Ravish
Rajiv Keni, Sreekanta Swamy, M. Sowmya, Ryan Costa Silva, Ligia Peixoto, Joana Rosa Martins, Tânia
Vassalo, Inês Silva, Joana Rodrigues Santos, Imtiaz A. A. Chaudhry, Bushra I. Goraya, Arshia Riaz,
João Fernandes Seròdio, Catarina Favas, José Delgado Alves, Miguel Trindade, Luiza Rusu

Notice
Statements and opinions expressed in the chapters are these of the individual contributors and not
necessarily those of the editors or publisher. No responsibility is accepted for the accuracy of
information contained in the published chapters. The publisher assumes no responsibility for any
damage or injury to persons or property arising out of the use of any materials, instructions, methods
or ideas contained in the book.

First published in London, United Kingdom, 2022 by IntechOpen
IntechOpen is the global imprint of INTECHOPEN LIMITED, registered in England and Wales,
registration number: 11086078, 5 Princes Gate Court, London, SW7 2QJ, United Kingdom
Printed in Croatia

British Library Cataloguing-in-Publication Data
A catalogue record for this book is available from the British Library

Additional hard and PDF copies can be obtained from orders@intechopen.com

Giant-Cell Arteritis
Edited by Imtiaz A. Chaudhry
p. cm.
Print ISBN 978-1-83969-208-6
Online ISBN 978-1-83969-209-3
eBook (PDF) ISBN 978-1-83969-210-9

We are IntechOpen,
the world's leading publisher of
Open Access books
Built by scientists, for scientists

6,000+
Open access books available

148,000+
International authors and editors

185M+
Downloads

156
Countries delivered to

Our authors are among the

Top 1%
most cited scientists

12.2%
Contributors from top 500 universities

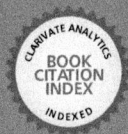

Interested in publishing with us?
Contact book.department@intechopen.com

Numbers displayed above are based on latest data collected.
For more information visit www.intechopen.com

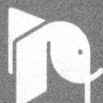

Meet the editor

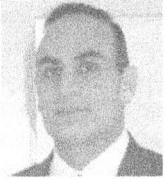

Dr. Imtiaz A. Chaudhry received his MD Ph.D. from the University of Utah School of Medicine and an internship and residency in ophthalmology from Yale University School of Medicine followed by a fellowship in ophthalmic plastic and reconstructive surgery from Baylor College of Medicine, Texas. Dr. Chaudhry spent 10 years as a full-time staff member and chief of oculoplastics and orbital surgery at King Khaled Eye Specialist Hospital, one of the largest eye hospitals in the Middle East. Since 2012, he has been the medical director for Houston Oculoplastics, Texas. He is on the active staff of the Houston Methodist Hospital, Memorial Hermann Hospital, Baylor St. Luke's Medical Center, and Texas Children's Hospital in Houston, Texas. He is also an adjunct professor of Ophthalmology at the Ruiz Department of Ophthalmology and Visual Sciences, The University of Texas- McGovern Medical School. Dr. Chaudhry is a skilled ophthalmic and facial plastic surgeon who has worked with patients from around the world. He specializes in cosmetic and reconstructive surgery of the eyelids and orbits and ophthalmic plastic and reconstructive surgery. He has experience working with patients who have suffered from acquired defects as well as those who have congenital defects of the eyelid and orbital-facial region. He is actively involved in teaching medical students, residents, and fellows. Over the past 20 years, Dr. Chaudhry has helped in training more than 100 ophthalmology residents and 10 fellows in oculoplastic surgery. In addition to his enormous skills in patient care, Dr. Chaudhry has extensive research, teaching, and leadership experience in the field of ophthalmology. Because of his contribution to the advancement of knowledge in this field, the American Academy of Ophthalmology honored him with the prestigious "Achievement Award" in 2008. His work in the field of ophthalmic plastic and reconstructive surgery has been presented domestically and internationally, and he has taught several courses at the World Ophthalmology Congress and the American Academy of Ophthalmology. He has authored and co-authored 200 journal articles, abstracts, and book chapters in ophthalmology.

Contents

Preface

Giant cell arteritis (GCA) is a systemic vasculitis that affects medium- to large-sized arteries, in which the inflammatory reaction destroys the artery wall with the fragmentation of the elastic lamina. Such phenomena can result in vision loss if not treated promptly. Other non-ocular symptoms noted include GCA, headache, tenderness in the temporal area of the scalp, myalgias and arthralgias, fever, weight loss, and jaw claudication. Clinical suspicion is an essential pathway to the diagnosis of this disease. Thus, immediate Westergren sedimentation rate and C-reactive protein should be obtained. A temporal artery biopsy, however, remains the most definitive diagnostic tool to support the clinical diagnosis of GCA. The incidence of GCA remarkably increases with each decade of age among those aged 50 years or older.

In Chapter 1, "Epidemiological Aspects of Giant Cell Arteritis", Riaz et al. discuss notable differences among patients of different ethnicities. They report that the epidemiological characteristics of GCA have been primarily researched in populations from the United States as well as several European countries with an emphasis on the Caucasian population. In more recent years, a handful of studies have emerged from non-European countries regarding the epidemiology of GCA. The results of these findings are in parallel with previous observations, which presumed GCA to be more common in European and North American populations. Nordic countries present the highest annual incidence rates of GCA, which moderately affects southern European countries (Italy, Spain, France, etc.). The lowest incidence rates have been reported in East Asian countries. The authors contend that diverse ethnical populations in countries such as the United States lead to variations across regions, such as a higher incidence rate in the Northern states due to Scandinavian ancestry. Different ethnicities present varying susceptibility, which may exhibit different degrees of suspicion with certain races, leading to influence on the number of biopsies performed and diagnoses made. In some regions, race and ethnicity is self-identified, which may reveal limited information on genetic background. The authors detail the varied incidence rate observed in different populations across the globe. The incidence rate increases substantially with age and a greater ratio of patients are women in most regions, except for Asian countries. Whether female susceptibility is genuinely lower in that region or whether this discrepancy is due to different health-seeking behavior is unknown. Although seasonal and cyclic patterns were observed in a few studies and environmental factors were suggested, such influence remains inconclusive. The authors also note that the definition of GCA is inconsistent across the literature, resulting in the inclusion of heterogeneous data during an extensive review. Hence, there may be an over- or underestimation of statistical values. The criteria for the diagnosis of this disease substantially varied, with incidence rates presented based on biopsy-proven cases, ACR criteria-fulfilling cases, or unspecified clinical diagnoses. Therefore, data may vary depending on which inclusion criteria were used. Moreover, the technicality for biopsy-proven cases (length of the segment or threshold for diagnosis) may also alter the rate of incidence. In many reviews, the length of the arterial specimen remains unmentioned. In 2016, an alteration to the list of criteria for a more comprehensive diagnosis of GCA was submitted.

In Chapter 2, "Cellular and Molecular Characteristics of Vascular Damage in Giant Cell Arteritis, the 'Unmet Needs' for Targeted Treatment", Rusu reports that GCA is a primary systemic vasculitis characterized by systemic inflammation and vascular insufficiency of large and medium blood vessels that may lead to end-organ damage in patients aged 50 years or older. Standard corticosteroid treatment of the disease significantly improves the intima-media thickness while having less influence on vascular endothelial dysfunction. The author describes that GCA morbidity may be related to both cardiovascular complications and corticosteroid toxicity. He discusses characteristic aspects of vascular damage and the several mechanisms that cause vascular dysfunction, intima-media "nodular" thickness, progressive narrowing of the arterial lumen, and vascular blockage in the context of systemic inflammation, thrombosis, and of cardiovascular complications in GCA along with new therapeutic glucocorticosteroid-sparing agents preventing life-threatening cardiovascular complications of GCA. Vasculitis is a heterogeneous group of conditions characterized by inflammation of the vessel wall resulting in narrowing or occlusion of the vessel lumen. The author emphasizes that the use of biomarkers in laboratory testing for GCA may become highly valuable once some specific diagnostic or prognostic blood biomarkers become available. Currently, the criteria used to diagnose GCA are the elevated inflammatory markers usually associated with ischemic events such as acute phase reactants frequently having high blood levels: ESR and CRP, elevated platelets and white blood cell numbers, and elevated blood von Willebrand factor. In addition, elevated serum level of the proinflammatory cytokine interleukin 6 (IL6) is critical in GCA pathogenesis and perhaps the most sensitive marker in GCA. The author emphasizes the role of glucocorticosteroid therapy since such treatment improves GCA symptoms immediately, especially in ischemic complications when it is lifesaving or avoids permanent invalidity (partial/total visual loss). Prompt treatment results in the improvement of blood supply to the vital organs, decreasing cerebrovascular events and myocardial infarction and improving vision loss. Because of the risk of acute CVA and visual loss, GCA is considered an ophthalmological emergency for which the treatment is high-dose methylprednisolone pulse therapy. In this review study, the authors discuss several cellular and molecular pathogenetic mechanisms of vascular damage characteristic of GCA that might occur during the progression of the disease, especially during the active phase. The paradigm in terms of GCA physiopathology is that inflammation starts in the adventitial layer with the activation of the vascular dendritic cells (DCs), which shifts the situation to the point where there are multiple types of immune cells recruited, proliferating, and differentiating in the vessel wall, causing together with inflamed vascular cells an erroneous repair of the arterial wall. It is unlikely that DCs are the cells driving these processes, given the multitude of cell functions the arterial wall's endothelial cells (ECs) play in complicated processes of vascular inflammation, hemostasis/ thrombosis, and vascular repair, resulting in a distinct GCA-specific vasculopathy most commonly referred to as GCA-related vascular remodeling. There are three EC populations in the GCA artery: arterial luminal ECs, vasa vasorum ECs, and capillary ECs formed de novo in the intima and media layers (which showed to be avascular in normal arteries) of the diseased artery. These three types of ECs are activated in a sequential manner; their activation is probably subordinated to the invading immune cells, but not to all. For instance, vasa vasorum ECs are activated after vascular DCs are activated, but ECs activation most probably precedes the activation of T cells. The invading cells must get into the vessel wall through the vasa vasorum. Activated ECs provide the means for invasion by mobilizing, performed contents of storage granules WPBs. These secreted ECs mediators are released in a timely manner to fulfill proinflammatory, chemoattractant, and neoangiogenic roles or increased endothelial permeability functions. GCA 18 biomarkers have the potential to detect the disease that is missed by TAB/imaging. Several large multi-center clinical trials have led to the discovery of new potential biomarkers to monitor disease activity and relapses, which is a new critical development in the field. Some of the recently published data imply that testing several blood acute phase reactants can optimize earlier diagnosis and the ability to predict flares and complications . In addition, our study underlines the importance of the candidate targets for novel therapeutics. In the more severe complications of this disease, such as blindness or stroke, the underlying GCA-related vascular damage does not respond to GS, as previously reported by several independent studies. A multi-step treatment for GCA should be envisioned that involves steroids, especially when people with GCA are particular ill, and efficient medication to control vascular dysfunction (e.g., to lower proinflammatory cytokine levels, to lower the levels of circulating active vWF in parallel). Of the variety of GCA treatments being investigated, a few have the potential to improve outcomes and reduce the need for steroids. The availability of the new drug tocilizumab was received with a lot of enthusiasm, as it is the only FDA-approved drug for GCA treatment. Tocilizumab is effective to control GCA symptoms, allowing rapid GS tapering, and persistent remission with a low dose GS after six months of follow-up; however, after tocilizumab discontinuation the relapse-free survival percentage decreases, at least in some patients. Tocilizumab poses certain challenges for clinicians regarding biomarker follow-up of patients, since the drug represses both CRP and ESR, thus making careful anamnesis, physical examination, and clinical judgment even more important for disease assessment. Twenty adverse events were considered directly related to the drug; danger with tocilizumab administration was reported in the instance of infection in patients receiving tocilizumab, with pneumonia and no CRP and ESR rise, signifying that more careful assessing of disease activity and infections in patients treated with tocilizumab is required. Further studies are needed to determine the optimal duration of treatment and maintaining of dosing and to further reduce the risk of relapse. An important note to make is that molecular pathogenic pathways promoting GCA disease are changing as the disease progresses under treatment. This situation is frequent in clinical practice and requires adequate follow-up and adapted therapeutic strategies. Hopefully, future research will bring us closer to the goal of identifying new therapies for active and/or refractory GCA, which used in substitution or addition to steroids will provide tide control of the disease, addressing not only vascular inflammation but also vascular remodeling, skewed thrombotic propensity, and luminal changes in GCA patients at risk of VL, stroke, or other ischemic events at the initial onset of the arterial disease or in evolution.

Recent advances in imaging studies and treatment approaches have greatly improved our knowledge of GCA. Previously thought of as a predominantly cranial disease, we now know that GCA is a systemic disease that may involve other medium and large vessel territories. Several imaging studies have shown that between 30% and 70% of patients with GCA present with large-vessel vasculitis. Moreover, a significant proportion of patients present large-vessel disease in the absence of cranial involvement. GCA is commonly defined as Large-Vessel (LV) GCA if the aorta and its branches are involved. The extra-cranial disease also poses management challenges, as these patients may have a more refractory-relapsing disease course and need additional therapies. Aortic dilation and aneurysms are well-described late complications of GCA involving the large artery territories.

In Chapter 3 "Extra-Cranial Involvement in Giant Cell Arteritis", Serodio, Trinadade, Favas, and Alves discuss the clinical picture of extra-cranial involvement in GCA, focusing on improved diagnostic protocols and suitable treatment strategies. The authors mention that in the past LV-GCA has been mis-regarded and underdiagnosed. They note that in recent years there has been an increased awareness of the systemic larger artery nature of GCA, based on necropsy studies that have shown histologic evidence of systemic large-artery vasculitis in approximately 80% of patients. Recent advances in diagnostic imaging techniques have confirmed these figures, suggesting that imaging will have an increasing impact on the diagnosis and management of GCA. Furthermore, patients with GCA are at increased risk of developing aortic dilation and aneurysms, among other complications. Altogether, these issues highlight the importance of the extra-cranial involvement of GCA, which has been under-recognized and poorly managed. The interaction of immunopathogenic mechanisms with the different functional and anatomic characteristics of the vessel walls in different parts of the body may explain the distinct aspects of LV-GCA pathophysiology. The authors state that there is consistent evidence confirming that arteries are involved in around two-thirds of patients with GCA and one-third of patients with PMR. Classification criteria are inadequate for LV-GCA and thus a revision of the current criteria may be needed soon. The authors believe that LV-GCA presents a more relapsing-disease course and an increased risk of vascular complications, with LV inflammation being responsible for a considerable increase in the morbidity and mortality associated with this condition. This chapter emphasizes the importance of carefully considering the large artery aspects in the management and treatment of patients with GCA.

The use of medical image processing and analysis tools have improved GCA detection and diagnosis using patient-specific medical imaging In Chapter 4, "Medical Image Processing and Analysis Techniques for Detecting Giant Cell Arteritis", Qasrawi, Al-Halawa, Daraghmeh, Hjouj, and Seir propose several image processing and analysis algorithms for detecting and quantifying GCA from patient medical images. They introduce the connected threshold and region growing segmentation approaches to two case studies with temporal arteritis using US and MRI imaging modalities extracted from a Radiopedia dataset. They developed a GCA detection procedure using the 3D Slicer Medical Imaging Interaction software as a fast prototyping, open-source framework. According to the authors, GCA detection passes through two main procedures: the pre-processing phase, in which the quality of an image is improved and enhanced after removing noise (irrelevant and unwanted parts of the scanned image) using filtering techniques and contrast enhancement methods; and the processing phase, which includes all the steps of processing used for identification, segmentation, measurement, and quantification of GCA. The semi-automatic interaction involves the entire segmentation process for finding the segmentation parameters. The results of two case studies in this chapter show that the proposed approach managed to detect and quantify the GCA region of interest. According to the authors, the proposed algorithm is efficient to perform complete and accurate extraction of temporal arteries. The proposed method can be used for studies focusing on 3D visualization and volumetric quantification of GCA. These algorithms depend on various image processing algorithms, including image enhancement, noise reduction, pixel densities histogram analysis, and statistical analysis tools. First, the Gaussian filters and noise reduction algorithms are applied to enhance the temporal artery structures, which effectively enhances the temporal artery contrast. Then, seed points are detected automatically through a threshold pre-processing operation. Based on the set of seed points and threshold analysis, region growing is applied, which grows in the target region. Then, the temporal artery region is extracted by connected threshold and region growing approaches, which can segment the artery due to the pixel intensity thresholds and the seed point approach. Three regions of interest can be extracted: the temporal artery wall, the blood flow, and the GCA region. Finally, the statistical and measurement tools are used to quantify the diameters, area, and volume of the GCA regions, and to detect and identify the size and location of the GCA region.

In Chapter 5, "Giant Cell Arteritis: From Neurologist's Perspective", Keni et al. discuss a detailed aspect of GCA that include risk factors, clinical symptoms and examination findings, investigations, treatment, and management of relapse. The authors emphasize having a detailed ophthalmological history and examination that includes aspects of transient or permanent visual loss, visual field defect, relative afferent pupillary defect, anterior ischemic optic neuritis, and central retinal artery occlusion. Some of the investigations the authors recommend in the evaluation of suspected GCA include complete blood count, renal function tests, liver function tests, CRP, and ESR. Some of the other investigations recommended are chest X-ray and urinalysis. Temporal artery biopsy remains the gold standard to support the clinical diagnosis of GCA. Negative biopsy results do not rule out the condition. The findings on temporal artery biopsy in GCA are characterized by inflammatory infiltration of the arterial wall by lymphocytes, macrophages, and giant cells in about 50% of cases. Color-coded duplex US can be utilized to examine the temporal, extracranial, occipital, and subclavian arteries, having a sensitivity of 85% and a specificity of more than 90%. The "halo sign" of the inflammatory edema of the vascular wall is visible as hypoechoic wall thickening is characteristic. Positron emission tomography (PET) uses radioactive metabolites to visualize metabolic processes. Spatial resolution is limited with PET, so visualization can only be determined in the aorta and larger vessels, and the ability to visualize the temporal arteries is limited. However, MRI may be useful as the imaging modality for temporal arteries. Detailed imaging of the walls and lumen of the temporal artery is possible by doing a high-resolution MRI (fat suppression, T1 weighted). Diagnosis of GCA is based on clinical and laboratory tests. In cases where there is a clinical suspicion of GCA, corticosteroid treatment should be initiated immediately and not delayed awaiting the results of blood tests or temporal artery biopsy. In cases of complicated GCA, when there is evolving visual loss or amaurosis fugax, intravenous methylprednisolone in a dosage of 500 mg–1 g IV for three days followed by oral prednisone in the dose range of 40–60 mg daily with a tapering regimen is recommended. In cases of relapse, a rise in inflammatory markers (ESR/CRP) is usually seen, however, these markers can remain normal in some cases. The use of secondary agents such as methotrexate or azathioprine should be considered in patients with recurrent relapse or failure. Clinical experience has shown that methotrexate (7.5–15 mg once a week) reduces the relapse rate and overall duration of exposure to corticosteroids. Tocilizumab is an interleukin-6 (IL-6)-receptor inhibitor. The GCA Actemra (GiACTA) trial demonstrated increased rates of sustained remission using a combination of tocilizumab plus corticosteroids compared to treatment with corticosteroids alone. Furthermore, steroid-induced adverse effects have been reduced with the usage of tocilizumab. Tocilizumab is recommended by NICE as an option for treating GCA in adults if they have relapsing or refractory disease and they have not already taken tocilizumab; it is stopped after one year of uninterrupted treatment at most. Tocilizumab is a potent suppressor of IL-6, which is an important producer of CRP. Therefore, patients on tocilizumab may not produce a biochemical inflammatory response in the setting of infection/inflammation. Caution should be taken while taking tocilizumab, particularly in patients with a history of diverticulitis, as it carries a risk for gastrointestinal perforation.

In Chapter 6, "Clinical Manifestations of Giant Cell Arteritis", Silva, Silva, Santos, Vassalo, Martins, and Peixoto discuss the clinical manifestations of GCA in detail. They report that GCA is commonly categorized as a large- and medium-sized vessel vasculitis with systemic symptoms being common. Systemic symptoms associated with GCA are frequent and include fever, fatigue, anorexia, and weight loss. These symptoms may occur for a few days and may prolong to several weeks. Fever is usually low grade and occurs in up to one-half of patients. It has been stated as well that 1 out of 6 fevers of unknown origin in older adults may have been due to GCA. About 10% of patients with GCA present with constitutional symptoms and laboratory evidence of inflammation as the only clues to the diagnosis. Headache is a common presentation of GCA, being the initial symptom in 33% of cases and present in about 80% of patients, which is either new in a patient without previous history of headaches or of a new type in a patient with chronic headaches. Headaches due to GCA are typically throbbing and continuous, located over the temples, but can also be frontal, occipital, unilateral, or generalized. Descriptions of the pain range from a dull or burning sensation to focal tenderness on direct palpation. Patients may note scalp tenderness with hair combing or when wearing a hat. Jaw claudication results from ischemia of the maxillary artery supplying the masseter muscles and is highly predictive of temporal arteritis. Nearly 50% of patients experience jaw claudication, a symptom consisting of mandibular pain, discomfort, or fatigue triggered by mastication or prolonged speaking and relieved by stopping. The incidence of permanent loss of vision ranges from 15% to 20% of patients. When untreated, contralateral eye involvement commonly occurs within the first two weeks after initial onset. Extraocular motility disorders occur in approximately 5% of patients and include diplopia, which has a high specificity when accompanied by other symptoms suggestive of GCA. Diplopia, which is usually transient, can result from ischemia of any portion of the oculomotor system, including the brainstem, oculomotor nerves, and the extraocular muscles themselves. Less common manifestations reported include CNS involvement, audiovestibular and upper respiratory symptoms, pericarditis, mesenteric ischemia, and female genital tract involvement. Patients with GCA are at increased risk for pulmonary and cardiovascular events, but cardiac involvement is rare. Stroke is a rare but important complication of GCA and is typically due to stenosis of the carotid and the vertebral or basilar arteries. Even with aggressive steroids and immunosuppressive therapy, it is associated with high morbidity and mortality. More than one-half of strokes attributable to GCA occur in the vertebrobasilar system. Bilateral vertebral artery involvement, which causes rapidly progressive brainstem or cerebellar neurologic deficits with high mortality, is highly suggestive of GCA. Peripheral neuropathy, myelopathy, higher cortical dysfunction or dementia, and pachymeningitis are uncommon complications of GCA. GCA is closely linked to polymyalgia rheumatica (PMR) and this well-known association has therapeutic and prognostic consequences. About 40% to 60% of GCA patients have manifestations of PMR, an inflammatory rheumatic condition clinically characterized by symmetrical proximal polyarthralgia and myalgia, with aching and stiffness on shoulders, hip girdle, neck, torso, and an unfamiliar sense of fatigue. Less commonly, distal findings can occur, involving synovitis of peripheral joints, especially at the wrists and metacarpophalangeal joints, with distal extremity swelling and pitting edema, known as remitting seronegative symmetrical synovitis with pitting edema (RS3PE) syndrome, puffy edematous hand syndrome, or distal extremity swelling with pitting edema. The authors emphasize that GCA should always be considered in the differential diagnosis of a new-onset headache in patients 50 years of age or older with an elevated ESR. The onset of symptoms in GCA tends to be subacute, but abrupt presentations occur in some patients. Although systemic manifestations are characteristic of GCA, vascular involvement can be widespread. Clinical manifestations of the disease most frequently result from the involvement of the cranial branches of arteries originating from the aortic arch. A complete diagnosis of GCA requires the presence of American College of Rheumatology (ACR) classification modified criteria: a. age over 50 years at the onset of the disease; b. moderate, bitemporal, recently installed headache; c. scalp tenderness, abnormal temporal arteries on inspection and palpation, reduced pulse, jaw claudication; d. blurred vision or permanent visual loss in one or both; e. systemic symptoms (fatigue, weight loss, fever, pain in the shoulders and hips: polymyalgia rheumatica); f. increased inflammatory markers (ESR > 50 mm/h, CRP > 1.5 mg/dl); g. representative histologic findings on TAB: mononuclear cell infiltration or granulomatous inflammation of the vessel wall, usually accompanied with multinucleated giant cells. Several imaging techniques may be suitable for the diagnosis of GCA. Compared to other imaging techniques, the US is the most suitable for the evaluation of GCA patients. The test can easily be performed by the clinician usually immediately after the general examination of the patient, and it significantly shortens the waiting period until another investigation is performed. Ultrasonography is a safe, non-invasive, accessible, fast, and low-cost bedside screening technique that has the unique capacity of studying real-time hemodynamics. It presents the ability to evaluate the anatomy of a vessel's wall, identifying equally parietal abnormalities (wall thickening, hypoechoic plaques, clotting, parietal hematoma, dissections) and the external diameter of the artery; it can rule out both stenosis and occlusion. The use of US is widespread in neurological clinical practice, mainly in the evaluation of arterial atherosclerotic process but also for monitoring other diseases such as medium-/large-vessel vasculitis. The advantages of US over other imaging techniques in GCA are represented by its safety, accessibility, tolerability, speed, and high resolution (a high-frequency probe offers both an axial and a lateral resolution of 0.1 mm. The smaller the vessel diameter, the more difficult is to appreciate the vessel wall damages, so that, in this case, the most informative US data are based on Doppler spectral evaluation. This is also valid for the assessment of medium- to small-vessel inflammation such as intracranial vasculitis. Using the US, one can reveal pathological characteristics in GCA: non-compressible arteries (compression sign), wall thickening ("halo" sign), stenosis, and vessel occlusion. There are three important items in the US diagnosis of temporal arteritis: "dark halo" sign, a typically homogeneous, hypoechoic, circumferential wall thickening around the lumen of an inflamed TA, which represents vessel wall edema, and a characteristic finding in temporal arteritis/GCA.

In Chapter 7, "An Integrated Approach to the Role of Neurosonology in the Diagnosis of Giant Cell Arteritis", Jianu, Jianu, Munteanu, Dan, Gogu, and Petrica discuss the importance of US in the diagnosis of TA. The authors emphasize that the US should be used as a first-line diagnostic investigation for patients presenting with clinical and biological features suggestive for GCA, taking into consideration that it has a high sensitivity to detect vessel wall thickening (dark halo sign) in the case of large/medium vessels. In their practice, CCDS has emerged as a safe and reliable alternative to TAB as a point-of-care diagnostic tool in the management of temporal arteritis. Because findings of TAs in the US do not correlate with eye complications in GCA, CDI of the orbital vessels is of critical importance to quickly differentiate the mechanism of eye involvement. The authors believe that the US may be helpful to detect the blood flow in the orbital vessels, especially in cases of the opacity of the medium or when the clinical appearance of ophthalmologic complications in temporal arteritis is atypical. The spectral Doppler analysis of the orbital vessels in GCA with eye involvement reveals low blood velocities, especially EDV, and high RI in all orbital vessels, in both orbits, for all patients (especially on the affected side). An added advantage of CDI of orbital vessels is that it provides immediate information that can be used to make treatment decisions, including a potential reduction in loss of sight and avoidance of unnecessary long-term steroid treatment by early exclusion of mimics. US has a high sensitivity to detect vessel wall thickening in the case of large vessel GCA. The eye involvement in GCA is frequent and consists of A-AION or CRAO, with abrupt, painless, and severe loss of vision of the involved eye. Because findings of TA's and the US do not correlate with eye complications in GCA, color Doppler imaging of the orbital vessels is of critical importance. Doppler US reveals low-end diastolic velocities and high resistance index to quickly differentiate the mechanism of eye involvement (A-AION versus N-AION). A-AION should be treated promptly with systemic corticosteroids to prevent further visual loss of the fellow eye.

Imtiaz A. Chaudhry, MD Ph.D. FACS
Medical Director,
Houston Oculoplastics,
Adjunct Professor,
Ruiz Department of Ophthalmology and Visual Sciences,
The University of Texas- McGovern Medical School,
Houston, Texas, USA

Chapter 1

Epidemiological Aspects of Giant Cell Arteritis

Arshia Riaz, Bushra I. Goraya and Imtiaz A. Chaudhry

Abstract

Giant cell arteritis (GCA) is a systemic vasculitis that affects medium-to-large-sized arteries, in which the inflammatory reaction destroys the artery wall with the fragmentation of the elastic lamina. Such phenomena can result in vision loss if not treated promptly. Other nonocular symptoms noted include GCA, headache, tenderness in the temporal area of the scalp, myalgias and arthralgias, fever, weight loss, and jaw claudication. Clinical suspicion is an essential pathway to the diagnosis of this disease. Thus, immediate Westergren sedimentation rate and C-reactive protein should be obtained. A temporal artery biopsy, however, remains the most definitive diagnostic tool. The incidence of GCA remarkably increases with each decade of age among those aged 50 years or over. Additionally, there have been notable differences among patients of different ethnicities. The epidemiological characteristics of GCA have been primarily researched in populations from the United States as well as several European countries with emphasis on the Caucasian population. In more recent years, a handful of studies have emerged from non-European countries regarding the epidemiology of GCA. The results of these findings are in parallel with previous observations, which presumed GCA to be more common in European and North American populations.

Keywords: giant cell arteritis, epidemiology, visual loss, temporal artery biopsy, incidence rate

1. Introduction

The first account of giant cell arteritis (GCA) can be traced back to tenth-century Baghdad by Arab ophthalmologist of medieval Islam Ali ibn Isa al-Kahhal. It was then more precisely described by Sir Jonathan Hutchinson in 1890, who noted the peculiar thrombotic appearance of the temporal artery (TA), a defining feature of the course of GCA. With the progression of the discovery of this disease and various case studies exploring its nature, ophthalmologists have additionally attempted to view how GCA could affect certain populations. During the second half of the twentieth century and the course of the twenty-first century, facilities across continents have published their findings on the tendencies of GCA to affect certain individuals more than others. In this chapter, we describe the epidemiology of GCA across continents and countries from individual reports and studies presenting the incidence rate of this vasculitis in their respective locations or populations.

2. Europe

Europe remains the continent with the most abundant publications pertaining to the epidemiology of GCA. One of the longest studies on the epidemiology of GCA was conducted in Western Norway, a retrospective study encompassing cases from 1972 to 2012 [1]. This study was one among many that noted how changing the criteria for the identification of GCA could greatly alter its incidence, especially due to the rarity of this vasculitis. For instance, the incidence rate of patients potentially affected by GCA satisfying the ACR 1990 criteria was 16.7 per 100,000 persons over 50 years of age. The incidence of patients clinically diagnosed as having GCA was 18.4 per 100,000 persons aged 50 years or more. Meanwhile, the incidence of biopsy-proven GCA was 11.2 per 100,000 persons over 50 years of age. The extended period of this study additionally contributed to the lowering of the mean annual incidence. When solely evaluating cases during a certain 5-year period (from 1992 to 1996), the incidence rate was found to be 26.7 per 100,000 persons over 50 years of age. Regardless of this, the prevalence remained among the highest recorded globally. This study also describes the increasing GCA incidence with age, where an older individual has a greater susceptibility to acquiring this vasculitis, as well as a greater ratio of women having this disease. Similarly, in the southern region of Norway, comparisons with past records from the same set of population were provided [2]. In a study spanning a period of 14 years (2000–2013), the Hospital of Southern Norway presented a GCA occurrence rate of 16.8 per 100,000 persons over the age of 50 years, one of the highest recorded globally and in line with other epidemiological findings from the Scandinavian region. As previously noted, one must consider that a small study sample and a short study period both have the potential of overestimating the incidence of a disease, as demonstrated by this study. In the same vicinity, the rate of giant cell arteritis in Western Nyland, Finland was examined [3]. From 1984 and 1988, 54 patients were diagnosed with GCA, among which 16 patients had a positive biopsy. The retrospective annual incidence of GCA was 69.8 for every 100,000 individuals older than 50 years. From 1984 to 1990, 133 patients in Iceland fulfilling the ACR criteria for GCA were identified, rendering an incidence rate of 27 in 100,000 people older than 50 years [4]. This study also suggests that the clinicians' greater tendency to suspect GCA and perform TA biopsies (TABs) may have contributed to a higher statistical incidence. The results of these studies and their reported high mean annual incidence rates go on to highlight the possibility of a greater susceptibility to GCA among Scandinavian population. These are among the highest globally, supporting the claim that the Scandinavian population is most considerably afflicted by this inflammatory disease.

When gauging the incidence of GCA cases in other parts of Europe, we witness a lowering in the number of cases. For instance, in Italy, 285 cases of biopsy-proven GCA were observed in the Reggio Emilia area from 1986 to 2012 [5]. The adjusted incidence rate was 5.8 per 100,000 people older than 50 years of age and was significantly greater in women. In Lugo, Spain, a retrospective study was conducted from 1986 to 1995 to identify the occurrence rate of biopsy-proven GCA [6]. The mean annual incidence was computed for each 5-year period, rendering a rate of 8.26 and 10.49 per 100,000 people older than 50 years, respectively. Nearby countries and regions in the southern part of Europe presented similar incidence rates, demonstrating the moderate tendency of individuals from this area of the continent of being acquiring GCA. Namely, the incidence rate in France was concluded to be between 7 and 10 individuals out of 100,000 older than 50 years [7]. Likewise, in Slovenia, the estimated annual incidence rates of GCA were overall 8.7 per 100,000 aged greater than 50 years. This lowered rate suggests a different ethnic make up in the region that is perhaps less susceptible to acquiring this vasculitis, suggesting a genetic factor, while the geographical location in a lower latitude than the Scandinavian region may imply an environmental etiology. The exact etiology remains unknown.

Epidemiological studies from 2002 to 2008 in Southern Europe and Northwestern Turkey aimed to assess the epidemiology of GCA by following patients at Trakya University Medical Faculty [8]. During this period, the incidence of GCA was found to be 1.13 patients per 100,000 persons 50 years of age or older. The incidence of GCA for females was slightly greater than that for males. The fact that this study relied on a single center presents the possibility of missing individuals who sought care in a different location or simply neglected their condition. Regardless of this, the contribution of this report is crucial due to the paucity of epidemiological outlook on GCA in this space.

3. Asia

A retrospective study of patients with giant cell arteritis in China was performed from August 1992 to May 2014 at the Peking Union Medical College Hospital [9]. A total of 70 patients were diagnosed with GCA. The demographic data of these patients differed from that in the previously discussed epidemiological studies in Europe. First, the average age of Chinese GCA patients was 65.2 years. This age at onset is lower than the mean reported age in other populations, which hovered between 70 and 80 years. In addition, male patients with GCA predominated the study, which differed from most reports globally. Chinese male may be more susceptible to GCA than female or they may present greater health-seeking behavior. It is important to note that patients in this study were identified from a single healthcare center, which may substantially underestimate the occurrence of this vasculitis despite its current rare occurrence. On a similar note, statistical records, pathology records, and case records from university hospitals were gathered to estimate an annual incidence of one out of 100,000 people aged older than 50 years in Hong Kong [10]. These findings suggest the particularly lower frequency of GCA among the Chinese population. In 1998, a nationwide survey was performed in Japan, revealing 690 patients treated for GCA in the previous year [11]. An incidence rate of the population was calculated to be 1.47 per 100,000 people older than 50 years of age. In conclusion, the epidemiological reports of GCA from East Asian countries reveal extremely low prevalence of GCA among this population.

From 2008 to 2014, a total of 17 patients fulfilling the classification criteria for GCA in India were identified [12]. Comparably to a previously discussed study in China, the mean age of GCA patients in the Indian population was 67 years, lower than the mean age from European reports. In addition, individuals with GCA in India were predominately male. The reasoning behind a lower mean age and a male predominant patient status is unknown and was hypothesized to be due to the greater likelihood of individuals with these characteristics to seek healthcare.

The rarity of GCA among the Indian population was demonstrated at Moorfields Eye Hospital, a center in London, UK [13]. From 2006 to 2014, patients of Indian descendance were significantly less likely to have a biopsy-positive GCA. Perhaps, some ethnicities are less likely to present a positive result to the TA biopsy or clinicians may simply be more likely to diagnose these individuals with GCA. A study of this nature, in which ethnicities are compared in a population, could provide important findings on the vulnerability of certain individuals to present with this vasculitis.

4. Middle east

The true incidence of GCA in the Arab population is difficult to assess due to the absence of a more nationwide perspective as well as a lack of population-based study in Arab countries. In a 22-year study, the epidemiology of GCA in Saudi Arabia was investigated [14]. From 1983 to 2004, 102 patients at King Khaled Eye Specialist Hospital underwent TAB, as seen in **Figure 1**, and seven patients were identified with biopsy-proven GCA. They noted that the incidence of GCA increases with age. Regardless of this, many aspects of the healthcare system in Saudi Arabia closely resemble that of the United States, with a similar life expectancy and a ratio of ophthalmologists relative to the size of the population.

In 1980, the incidence of giant cell arteritis in Jerusalem over a 25-year period was evaluated in a study involving four general hospitals in Jerusalem [15]. Among them, 170 patients with GCA had a positive TA biopsy. Furthermore, 36 biopsy-negative cases were also considered as they fulfilled the 1990 ACR criteria for GCA classification and responded adequately to steroid therapy. The age-adjusted incidence rate was computed to be 11.3 per 100,000 people $\geq$50 years of age for all incorporated GCA cases, but lower at 9.5 for the biopsy-proven cases. Moreover, this study observed seasonal patterns with a statistically insignificant rise in GCA diagnosis during the summer. The incidence rate of GCA in this study is comparable with those in other Mediterranean countries, with a less prominent frequency of female patients.

The results of a cohort of 114 patients who met the 2016 rACR criteria for the diagnosis of GCA and underwent TAB over a 10-year period in a tertiary center, Rassoul Akram Hospital, in Tehran, Iran were described [16]. This finding reflects the increase in GCA incidence with age. Although this study did not sufficiently provided a macroscopic account of the incidence and manifestation of GCA in a population, it was the first study performed in Iran assessing the intricacies of characterizing GCA and the discrepancies that may arise as a result of heterogeneous studies, especially due to the absence of definite criteria for the diagnosis of GCA.

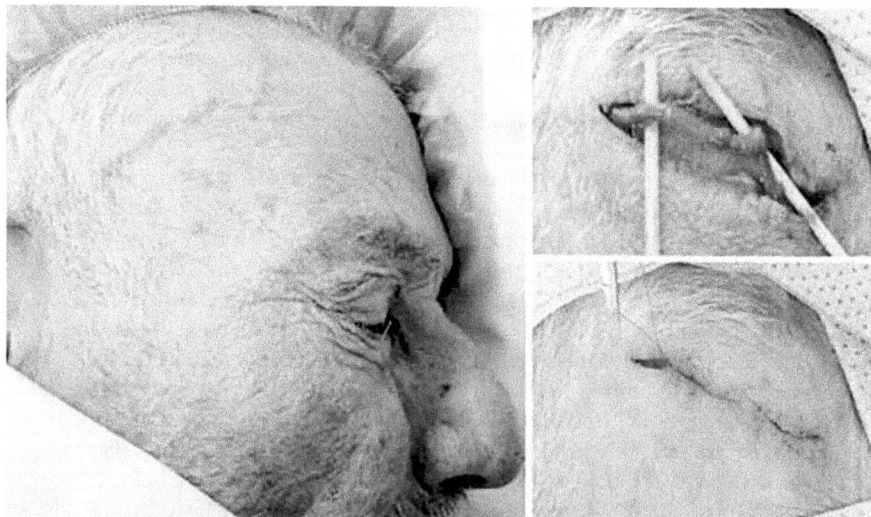

Figure 1.
A temporal artery biopsy involves acquiring a small section of the artery, which can potentially appear thrombotic. The length of the segment can vary across studies and may influence the results of the biopsy [14].

5. Africa

Africa stands out for its scarcity of information on GCA and its epidemiology. Perhaps, this could be due to an underdeveloped healthcare system, which hinders the proper equipment and tools for an adequate diagnosis, which could ultimately serve as data to be studied on a larger scale. It may also be that the African population has a lower susceptibility to GCA. In addition, the life expectancy in Africa is lower, which could influence statistics related to a disease with an increased likelihood of manifesting at a later stage in life. Therefore, it can be hypothesized that this region presents with lower rates of this vasculitis. The two studies discussing the epidemiology of GCA in the African population both pertain to French-colonized islands. From 1991 to 2016, data from two pathology units in Martinique, West Indies were reviewed to discuss the features of cases of biopsy-proven giant cell arteritis [17]. The findings fortified the assumption that GCA is less prevalent in an African descent population. Nevertheless, the retrospective nature of the study and the exclusion of a biopsy-negative GCA may have led to an underestimation of cases of GCA.

In a retrospective study from La Reunion near the Southwest region of the Indian Ocean from 2005 to 2017, an incidence rate roughly 4–12 times lower than in most European countries was calculated [18]. An exact count was difficult to provide due to the presence of a diverse group of ethnicities in La Reunion, especially from regions of the world with a lower prevalence of GCA. A shorter life expectancy may contribute to a lower frequency of cases observed as GCA increases with age. Other characteristics were found to be analogous observations made in previous epidemiological studies.

6. North America

Studies conducted in the United States have the potential of presenting important findings due to the possibility of comparing and contrasting features of a disease between ethnicities. A retrospective study spanning 11 years was conducted in the Texas Gulf Coast. Twenty-seven out of 101,239 patients aged 40 years or older had GCA. Intriguingly, 13 of these patients were black females, rendering it a noteworthy aspect of this study in which a significantly greater proportion of patients with GCA were black individuals [19].

A report from a study spanning from 1971 to 1980 in Shelby County, Tennessee identified 26 cases of GCA [20]. The average annual incidence was computed to be 1.58 per 100,000 individuals older than 50 years of age. The predominant patient from this study was white and female. This study presents one of the lowest frequencies of GCA cases across the globe. This could partially be due to the racial makeup of this population, which has a high percentage of black residents. African descent population is assumed to present a lower incidence rate of GCA. Among other contributions to a low incidence rate such as a retrospective design as well as inconsistencies in the diagnosis criteria, this study urged the need to consider environmental factors as potential causes for the onset of the vasculitis, such as the climate, exposure to the sun, frequency of rainfall, elevation, etc.

In another region of the United States, Olmsted County, Minnesota holds a population with northern European ancestry, which appears to be the group of people most severely afflicted by GCA. Therefore, the observation of a greater incidence rate may indicate a genetic factor in the onset of GCA. Between 1950 and 1991, 125 Olmsted County inhabitants were diagnosed with giant cell arteritis. The incidence per 100,000 persons 50 years of age or older was 17.8, which was significantly higher in women than in men. The incidence of GCA had increased to 19.8 from 2000 to 2009. The annual incidence rates substantially increased over the study period and with congregated cases of GCA, suggesting a regular cyclic pattern over time, which suggested the possibility of an infectious root for giant cell arteritis.

Previous studies suggested a low incidence of GCA in black patients, although conclusions were drawn from relatively small sample sizes. Nevertheless, the impression that GCA rarely impacts black individuals is generally assumed. Some reports have sought to compare GCA more directly between two races. A multi-center study involving 10 healthcare institutions was conducted to evaluate the presentation of GCA in African Americans [21]. An African American group of patients was compared with a cohort of Caucasian patients with a positive biopsy for ophthalmic GCA. Both the groups appeared to have a similar sex distribution, as around 70% of patients in both the cohorts were females. At Johns Hopkins Wilmer Eye Institute, findings notably challenging the commonly held belief that GCA is uncommon in African Americans were presented [22]. However, annual rates may not be directly calculated due to racial distributions in patients not reflecting that of the census population of the city of Baltimore, a detail that needs to be approached diligently prior to establishing conclusions. Furthermore, the screening and diagnosis process may differ among races and ethnicities due to physicians and clinicians holding preconceived perception of a greater prevalence in certain populations.

When comparing the rate of GCA between Caucasians and Asians, a significant lower occurrence rate of GCA in Asians was identified, which they computed to be 0.26–3.8 per 100,000 individuals older than 50 years of age, in parallel with studies from Asia [23]. The data for this study were collected from the University of California San Francisco computer database for patients from July 1989 to July 2006.

Similarly, giant cell arteritis has been reported to be very rare in Hispanics. From 1996 to 2002, patients with GCA at the Bascom Palmer Eye Institute were assessed [24]. Rates of a positive temporal artery biopsy were similar among Hispanic and non-Hispanic patients. Thirty-two patients with biopsy-proven GCA revealed similar mean age, symptoms, and final visual acuity between Hispanic and non-Hispanic cohorts. Hispanic and non-Hispanic cases are similarly impacted by the onset of giant cell arteritis.

A retrospective review was performed of all the biopsy-positive cases of giant cell arteritis presenting to a neuro-ophthalmology practice in Saskatoon, Saskatchewan [2]. Records of 141 consecutive patients who underwent temporal artery biopsy at the Saskatoon Eye Centre from July 1998 to June 2003 were reviewed. The average age of the biopsy-positive patients was 76.5 years, and the patients were 2.4 times more likely to be women. A total of 35 patients had a European ancestry, while two patients were of Aboriginal descent. The estimated incidence of GCA for Saskatoon was 9.4 per 100,000 for people over the age of 50 years. This study reveals the prospect of GCA to affect the people of Aboriginal descent despite a probable low incidence rate.

7. South America

Very few studies pertaining to the epidemiology of GCA have come from South American countries. One that most closely attempted to depict the status of GCA nationwide collected findings from three university hospitals in Brazil for patients with GCA between 2009 and 2010 [25]. This was, in fact, the first study addressing the features of GCA in Brazilian patients having the disease. Most GCA patients were Caucasians, while a few were of a combined European and Indigenous lineage. The Caucasian cohort was mostly of Portuguese, Italian, or Spanish ancestry. These suggested the possibility of asymptomatic manifestations, which may skew the epidemiological perspective of this disease.

8. Oceania

The last geographic region to be discussed is Oceania, which can be hypothesized to most closely resemble findings from Europe. From 1992 to July 2011, 314 cases of biopsy-proven GCA in South Australia were studied, in which the incidence for people over the age of 50 was 3.2 per 100,000 individuals [26]. Most characteristics of the disease were in line with observations described in studies from Europe, including a similar mean age and female predominance. Seasonal variations were additionally perceived, with a greater amount of diagnosis occurring during the summer season.

Cyclical variations were similarly noted in a study conducted in Otago, New Zealand. Records of 363 consecutive patients who underwent temporal artery biopsy at Dunedin Hospital between 1996 and 2005 were reviewed, with biopsy-proven GCA diagnosed in 70 patients. The mean annual incidence of GCA in Otago for people older than 50 years was 12.73 per 100,000 persons ≥50 years of age [26].

9. Conclusion

Nordic countries present the highest annual incidence rates of GCA. This vasculitis moderately affects southern European countries (Italy, Spain, France, etc.). The lowest incidence rates have been reported in East Asia. The diverse ethnical populations in countries such as United States lead to variations across regions, such as a higher incidence rate in the Northern states due to Scandinavian ancestry. Different ethnicities may present varying susceptibility because clinicians may exhibit different degree of suspicion with certain races, leading to influence on the number of biopsies performed and diagnosis made. In some regions, race and ethnicity is self-identified, which may reveal limited information on genetic background. **Figure 2** reveals the varied incidence rate observed in different populations across the globe.

The incidence rate increases substantially with age and a greater ratio of patients are women in most regions, except for Asian countries. Whether female susceptibility is genuinely lower in that region or whether this discrepancy is due to different health-seeking behavior is unknown. Although seasonal and cyclic patterns were observed in a few studied and environmental factors were suggested, such influence remains inconclusive.

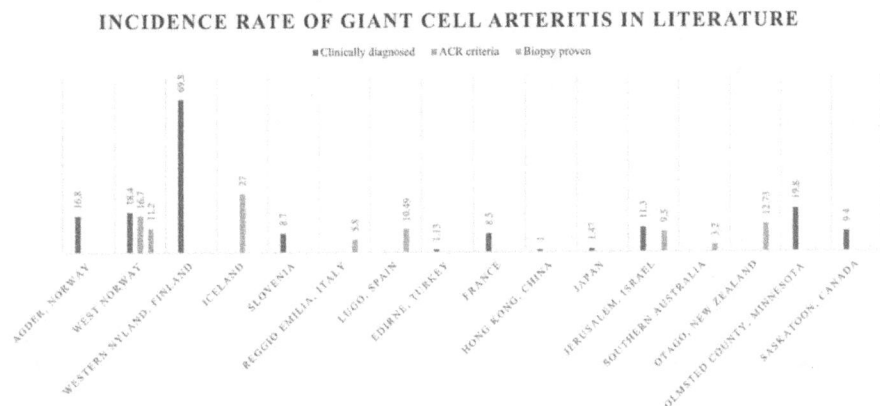

INCIDENCE RATE OF GIANT CELL ARTERITIS IN LITERATURE

Figure 2.
Graphical representation of incidence rates of GCA among some of the populations described in the literature. The highest incidence rates appear to be among the Scandinavian countries, regardless of the criteria utilized to diagnosis the incidence of GCA.

The definition of giant cell arteritis is inconsistent across literature, resulting in the inclusion of heterogeneous data during extensive review. Hence, there may be an over- or underestimation of statistical values. The criteria for the diagnosis of this disease substantially varied, with incidence rates presented based on biopsy-proven cases, ACR-criteria-fulfilling cases, or unspecified clinical diagnosis. Therefore, data may vary depending on which inclusion criteria were used.

Moreover, the technicality for biopsy-proven cases (length of the segment or threshold for diagnosis) may also alter the rate of incidence. In many reviews, the length of the arterial specimen remains unmentioned.

In 2016, an alteration to the list of criteria for a more comprehensive diagnosis of GCA was submitted. Furthermore, additional diagnostic tools have recently emerged, including the color Doppler ultrasound (CDUS), despite requiring extensive experience for utilization and a proper diagnosis. Other high-resolution magnetic resonance imaging technologies include magnetic resonance angiography (MRA), positron emission tomography (PET), computed tomography (CT), CT with angiography, and conventional MRA, which alternatively permit the visualization of the temporal artery. Although most reports attempted to thoroughly describe the equipment and tools for diagnosis, the heterogeneous approach across studies hinders appropriate comparisons, which may limit a precise epidemiological outlook of the disease in question.

Although this study repeatedly describes the rarity of GCA, it remains the most common vasculitis with severe consequences if remained untreated, ultimately resulting in permanent visual loss. Therefore, clinicians should remain diligent when coming across individuals presenting symptoms of the disease because an immediate course of action may greatly influence a person's course of life and impact their well-being physiologically and psychologically.

Author details

Arshia Riaz[1], Bushra I. Goraya[2] and Imtiaz A. Chaudhry[2*]

1 University of Texas, Austin, United States

2 Houston Oculoplastics, Houston, United States

*Address all correspondence to: orbitdr@yahoo.com

IntechOpen

References

[1] Brekke LK, Diamantopoulos AP, Fevang BT, Aβmus J, Esperø E, Gjesdal CG. Incidence of giant cell arteritis in Western Norway 1972-2012: A retrospective cohort study [published correction appears in Arthritis Res Ther. 2018 Dec 7;20(1):271]. Arthritis Research & Therapy. 2017;**19**(1):278

[2] Ramstead CL, Patel AD. Giant cell arteritis in a neuro-ophthalmology clinic in Saskatoon, 1998-2003. Canadian Journal of Ophthalmology. 2007;**42**(2): 295-298

[3] Franzén P, Sutinen S, von Knorring J. Giant cell arteritis and polymyalgia rheumatica in a region of Finland: An epidemiologic, clinical and pathologic study, 1984-1988. The Journal of Rheumatology. 1992;**19**(2):273-276

[4] Baldursson O, Steinsson K, Bjornsson J, Lie JT. Giant cell arteritis in Iceland. An epidemiologic and histopathologic analysis. Arthritis and Rheumatism. 1994;**37**(7):1007-1012

[5] Catanoso M, Macchioni P, Boiardi L, et al. Incidence, prevalence, and survival of biopsy-proven giant cell arteritis in northern italy during a 26-year period. Arthritis Care & Research (Hoboken). 2017;**69**(3):430-438

[6] Gonzalez-Gay MA, Miranda-Filloy JA, Lopez-Diaz MJ, Perez-Alvarez R, Gonzalez-Juanatey C, Sanchez-Andrade A, et al. Giant cell arteritis in northwestern Spain: A 25-year epidemiologic study. Medicine. 2007;**86**(2):61-68

[7] Mahr A, Belhassen M, Paccalin M, et al. Characteristics and management of giant cell arteritis in France: A study based on national health insurance claims data. Rheumatology (Oxford, England). 2020;**59**(1):120-128

[8] Pamuk ON, Dönmez S, Karahan B, Pamuk GE, Cakir N. Giant cell arteritis and polymyalgia rheumatica in northwestern Turkey: Clinical features and epidemiological data. Clinical and Experimental Rheumatology. 2009;**27**(5):830-833

[9] Sun F, Ma S, Zheng W, Tian X, Zeng X. A retrospective study of chinese patients with giant cell arteritis (GCA): Clinical features and factors associated with severe ischemic manifestations. Medicine (Baltimore). 2016;**95**(13):e3213

[10] Tam S, Wong TC. Temporal arteritis in Hong Kong. International Journal of Rheumatic Diseases. 2008;**11**:163-169

[11] Kobayashi S, Yano T, Matsumoto Y, et al. Clinical and epidemiologic analysis of giant cell (temporal) arteritis from a nationwide survey in 1998 in Japan: The first government-supported nationwide survey. Arthritis and Rheumatism. 2003;**49**(4):594-598

[12] Sharma A, Sagar V, Prakash M, et al. Giant cell arteritis in India: Report from a tertiary care center along with total published experience from India. Neurology India. 2015;**63**(5):681-686

[13] Tan N, Acheson J, Ali N. Giant cell arteritis in patients of Indian Subcontinental descent in the UK. Eye (London, England). 2019;**33**(3): 459-463

[14] Chaudhry IA, Shamsi FA, Elzaridi E, Arat YO, Bosley TM, Riley FC. Epidemiology of giant-cell arteritis in an Arab population: A 22-year study. The British Journal of Ophthalmology. 2007;**91**(6):715-718

[15] Bas-Lando M, Breuer GS, Berkun Y, Mates M, Sonnenblick M, Nesher G. The incidence of giant cell arteritis in Jerusalem over a 25-year period: Annual and seasonal fluctuations. Clinical and Experimental Rheumatology. 2007;**25** (1 Suppl 44):S15-S17

[16] Aghdam KA, Sanjari MS, Manafi N, Khorramdel S, Alemzadeh SA, Navahi RAA. Temporal artery biopsy for diagnosing giant cell arteritis: A ten-year review. Journal of Ophthalmic and Vision Research. 2020;**15**(2):201-209

[17] Moinet F, Molinie V, Polomat K, Merle H, Blettery M, Brunier-Agot L, et al. Biopsy proven giant cell arteritis in african descent populations: Incidence and characteristics in martinique, French West Indies. Arthritis & Rhematology. 2017;**69**(suppl 10):275-276

[18] Richier Q, Deltombe T, Foucher A, et al. AB0694 Giant cell arteritis epidemiology in la reunion: A retrospective cases series. Annals of the Rheumatic Diseases. 2018;**77**:1489

[19] Gonzalez EB, Varner WT, Lisse JR, Daniels JC, Hokanson JA. Giant-cell arteritis in the southern United States. An 11-year retrospective study from the Texas Gulf Coast. Archives of Internal Medicine. 1989;**149**(7):1561-1565

[20] Smith CA, Fidler WJ, Pinals RS. The epidemiology of giant cell arteritis. Report of a ten-year study in Shelby County, Tennessee. Arthritis and Rheumatism. 1983;**26**(10):1214-1219

[21] Garrity ST, Pistilli M, Vaphiades MS, et al. Ophthalmic presentation of giant cell arteritis in African-Americans. Eye (London, England). 2017;**31**(1):113-118

[22] Gruener AM, Poostchi A, Carey AR, et al. Association of giant cell arteritis with race. JAMA Ophthalmology. 2019;**137**(10):1175-1179

[23] Pereira LS, Yoon MK, Hwang TN, Hong JE, Ray K, Porco T, et al. Giant cell arteritis in Asians: A comparative study. The British Journal of Ophthalmology. 2011;**95**(2):214-216

[24] Lam BL, Wirthlin RS, Gonzalez A, Dubovy SR, Feuer WJ. Giant cell arteritis among Hispanic Americans. American Journal of Ophthalmology. 2007;**143**(1):161-163

[25] Souza AW, Okamoto KY, Abrantes F, Schau B, Bacchiega AB, Shinjo SK. Giant cell arteritis: A multicenter observational study in Brazil. Clinics (São Paulo, Brazil). 2013;**68**(3):317-322

[26] Dunstan E, Lester SL, Rischmueller M, et al. Epidemiology of biopsy-proven giant cell arteritis in South Australia. Internal Medicine Journal. 2014;**44**(1):32-39

Cellular and Molecular Characteristics of Vascular Damage in Giant Cell Arteritis, the 'Unmet Needs' for Targeted Treatment

Luiza Rusu

Abstract

Giant cell arteritis (GCA) is a primary systemic vasculitis characterized by systemic inflammation and vascular insufficiency of large and medium blood vessels which may lead to end-organ damage in patients age 50 and older. Standard corticosteroid treatment of GCA significantly improves the intima-media thickness while having less influence on vascular endothelial dysfunction. GCA morbidity may be related to both cardiovascular complications and corticosteroid toxicity. Therefore, we aim to discuss 1) characteristic aspects of vascular damage, 2) several mechanisms that cause vascular dysfunction, intima-media 'nodular' thickness, progressive narrowing of the arterial lumen and vascular blockage in the context of systemic inflammation, thrombosis and of the cardiovascular complications in GCA and 3) new therapeutic glucocorticosteroid-sparing (GS) agents which might be a more productive way of avoiding the invalidating or life-threatening cardiovascular complications of GCA.

Keywords: giant cell arteritis, mispositioned inflammation, vascular remodeling, von Willebrand factor, thrombosis, GS-saving therapeutic agents

1. Introduction

Vasculitis is a heterogenous group of conditions characterized by inflammation of the vessel wall resulting in narrowing or occlusion of the vessel lumen, aneurysm formation and impairment of downstream organ functions [1–3]. Vasculitis is classified according to the predominant size of the vessels involved into large, medium or small vessel vasculopathy [1–3].

Giant cell arteritis (GCA) is an autoimmune disease of the blood vessels, a disease where the immune system not only fails to protect but actively damages the blood vessels [4]. It is the most frequent primary vasculitis in adults. It manifests in patients mid age and older (odds 1:500 in this age group) [1]. The estimated annual incidence worldwide is 2.4 to 32.8 cases per 10^4 [3, 5]. GCA is a large-vessel vasculitis which has tropism for thoracic aorta and its extracranial branches [3, 6]. It affects mostly ethnic groups of northern European descent [7], especially female gender (3:1 ratio) [7, 8], and immune response polymorphisms associated with HLA-DRB1*04 alleles [9]. In a genome-wide association study collected from over 2000 GCA patients of European ancestry [9], two independent signals in the human leukocyte antigen MHC HLA II class region were reported recently to be strongly correlated with GCA [9]. Plasminogen and prolyl 4-hydroxylase subunit alpha 2 (an enzyme involved in collagen synthesis) have important roles in vascular damage and neoangiogenesis [9] and gene variants of both proteins are related to high GCA risk, suggesting a role of these factors in the underlying pathologic mechanisms of GCA [9]. The nongenetic etiopathogenesis of GCA is also not completely understood [1]. The role of environmental factors (the incidence of the disease increases seasonally) [7], viral (herpes-infected mice develop large vessel arteritis [10]) and bacterial infectious agents was reported [1, 7, 10].

The arterial adventitia (the external arterial layer where the GCA inflammation starts before it spreads inward) is rich in dendritic cells (DCs) [4]. These cells get activated by the interaction of their own toll-like receptors (TLRs) with pathogen-associated molecular patterns (PAMPs) [11]. Dendritic cells are immuno-surveillance cells which belong to the vessel wall, and, when activated, synthesize proinflammatory cytokines leading to activation of GCA pathogenic cascade [12–14]. To date and to our knowledge, no unique triggering pathogen has yet been singled out in GCA [1, 4].

GCA has a large spectrum of clinical manifestations [1], and many times it goes undiagnosed until a considerable amount of damage is done and complications occur [1]. People with GCA often are referred to several specialists: ophthalmologist (for partial/total visual loss), neurologist or ORL (for severe headaches and jaw pain), rheumatologist (polymyalgia reaction); when in fact GCA is a problem caused by inflammation in arteries of large and medium size [1, 6]. Ischemic complications of GCA and other systemic complications might be resulting in significant comorbidities and death [8]. If treated promptly and properly, the life expectancy does not change [15].

Temporal artery biopsy (TAB) is a gold standard for diagnosis of GCA [1]. TAB reliability might be reduced by the segmented pattern in which the lesions occur in the blood vessel [16, 17] and by longer time treatment (over 2 weeks) [1, 18].

Due to the fact that imaging testing might not be readily available, the use of biomarkers in laboratory testing for GCA is highly valuable but there are no specific diagnostic or prognostic blood biomarkers yet found for GCA [1]. The main criteria used to diagnose GCA are the elevated inflammatory markers [1] usually associated with for ischemic events. Acute phase reactants frequently have high blood levels: erythrocyte sedimentation rate (ESR) and more sensitive C-reactive protein (CRP), elevated platelets and white blood cell numbers, elevated blood von Willebrand factor (VWF) [1, 19, 20]; and in addition, GCA is associated with normocytic normochromic anemia [1]. Elevated serum level of the proinflammatory cytokine interleukin 6 (IL6) is critical in GCA pathogenesis and perhaps the most sensitive marker in GCA [21].

GCA is usually evaluated together with another related condition, polymyalgia rheumatica (PMR) [22]. PMR is not a vasculitis, but its relationship to GCA requires discussion because in some patients PMR evolves into GCA and 40–50% of GCA patients have polymyalgic symptoms [23]. In 20% of PMR patients with subacute presentation (proximal stiffness located in the shoulder area), abnormal blood work and high ESR and CRP, the disease will progress to GCA [22]. Imaging and pathology studies have shown subclinical arteritis may be much more common with PMR patients [18]. It is possible these two conditions represent two distinct phenotypes of the same pathological entity [23].

The standard therapy for GCA patients is glucocorticosteroid treatment [18] because it makes GCA symptoms better immediately, especially in ischemic complications when it is lifesaving or avoids a permanent invalidity (partial/total visual loss) [21]. For instance, heightened vascular inflammation progressively affects more vessels, compromising carotid vessels and other branches from aorta, that supply blood to vital organs (GCA-related cerebrovascular events [24, 25] and GCA-related myocardial infarction [26]) [8]. GCA affects the eye as well, and patients can have sudden and painless visual loss [27]. Because of the risk of progressive visual loss, GCA is an ophthalmology emergency for which the treatment is high-dose methylprednisolone pulse therapy (1000 mg i.v. for 3 days) within 24 h of the onset of GCA symptoms, which works as an effective 'emergency' treatment option to prevent evolving optic (and progressively central nervous system) [28] involvement [18]. If treatment is delayed more than 24 h, the blood supply to the eye can be cut off for enough time that restoration of vision might not occur. IV pulse therapy is followed with oral GS therapy [18].

In all, chronic administration of GS insures 90% of GCA patients will have GS-related side effects [29]. Therefore, a lot of research nowadays is focused on what treatment we can give instead of or in combination with GS to minimize side effects of GS in GCA, and in all the other types of vasculitis where we depend on GS for the immediate beneficial effects as well [30]. Ongoing clinical trial investigations are showing promising preliminary results. Most of the newer targets are not yet used in clinical practice because of toxicity, poor efficiency or because are under development, but nevertheless these biologics are key in deciphering the pathogenic mechanisms of GCA.

In this study we aim to (1) describe the characteristic aspects of vascular damage; (2) discuss several known mechanisms that cause vascular disfunction in GCA; (3) overview new therapeutic GS-sparing agents which might be a more productive way of avoiding the invalidating or life-threatening cardiovascular complications of GCA. We focus on the current knowledge updates about the GCA pathogenic mechanisms subsidiary to ischemic complications of the disease and their targeted treatment.

2. Characteristics of vascular damage in GCA arteries

Healthy arteries have a large lumen, the arterial wall histology comprises three distinct layers. The adventitia is the external layer, separated from the medial layer by the external elastic lamina, the medial muscular layer is separated from the internal layer by the internal elastic lamina and the intima is composed of unistratificated endothelial cells (ECs) [3]. Positive temporal artery biopsy (TAB) is the gold standard of GCA diagnosis [31], however due to the segmented pattern in which the lesions occur a TAB in a segment without lesion will generate a false negative GCA test. The typical histopathology of GCA arteries highlights transmural granulomatous inflammation. It consists of transmural mononuclear cell infiltration, mostly T cells, macrophages, numerous multinucleated giant cells (seen in 75% of cases), surrounded by low number B cells in all the layers of the artery [16]. The destruction of the internal elastic lamina, vascular smooth muscle cells (VSMCs) from the media to the intimal layer, and intima hyperplasia (IH) [1] are pathognomonic for GCA. IH protrudes in the lumen, progressively causing the occlusion of the vessel. Intraluminal thrombosis is reportedly seen in about 10–20% of GCA cases, probably occurring more frequently in the conditions of high shear in artery stenosis in GCA ischemic complications. A negative TAB does not exclude GCA [1].

The kind of inflammation pattern the vascular wall will take depends entirely on the initial injury events. In GCA, the site of inflammation is restricted the blood vessel wall [4, 11]. Typical GCA pathological findings involve local vascular inflammation, granulomatous infiltrate, and segmented lesions alternating with healthy segments [16]. GCA is characterized by a highly specific tropism to medium and large arteries of the upper extremities, neck and head in older people [1, 11, 32]. On the other hand, the fact that PMR and GCA have similar clinical presentation and a percentage of patients with GCA also have PMR suggest that these two clinical presentations might be two distinct phenotypes of the same pathological process [23].

Intriguingly, topography and histological structure dictate whether GCA lesions are likely to occur. GCA develops mainly in the 2nd-5th extracranial branches of the carotid arteries and upper extremities branches of the proximal aorta that have a highly visible internal elastic membrane and vasa vasorum. Temporal arteries are the most affected [1], and the vertebrobasilar [28] and the ophthalmic arteries can be affected as well [33]. Intracranial branches of the cervical arteries are small vessels that are not prone to GCA as their elastic membranes are very thin to inexistent and lack vasa vasorum because they are nourished through diffusion not through vasa vasorum [34, 35].

2.1 Vasculitis initial events

Under physiological conditions, the vascular wall mainly acts as a barrier between circulating immune cells and surrounding tissues. Besides its role in blood transport, blood gas regulation and preservation of wall integrity, the arterial network also has an immunosurveillance function [4]. The only immune cell known to be present in the healthy vascular wall is the intramural DCs, found in an immature state, characterized by the expression of C-C motif chemokine receptor 6 (CCR6) and a low density of Toll-like receptors (TLRs) [14].

Under pathological conditions, the large arteries turn into a target of autoimmune disease [4]. The main immunopathogenic mechanisms in the GCA arteries are progressing from the outside to the luminal side of the arterial wall, from the adventitia, where mural DCs reside, towards the intima [4].

2.1.1 The crucial role of dendritic cells in GCA pathogenesis

To date it is well known that DCs are the antigen-presenting cells (APCs)-belonging to the vessel wall-responsible for the initial steps in GCA pathogenesis [14]. Arteries use their wall-embedded sentinel cells, the dendritic cells (DCs) [14], to intervene and generate inflammatory responses [11]. This ability of large arteries to control localized and systemic inflammation using indigenous cell populations is a critical trigger element in this primary vasculitis [11, 12, 14]. Vascular DCs are mostly localized at adventitia/media border [12, 14]. In the presence of unknown, diverse, and non-specific PAMPs, resident DCs activate and break the "immune privilege" [4] in GCA arteries [12], DCs initiate the pathogenic cascade [11] and DCs sense the danger from a distance through PAMPs interactions with their specific toll-ligand-receptors (TLRs) [11]. In contrast to physiological conditions, in GCA arteries, activated DCs at the adventitial/media border fail to leave the artery lesion site, meaning they don't migrate to a lymph node, are retained in the granulomatous infiltrates in the wall of the arteries [14], amplifying a mispositioned inflammation reaction [14].

The TLR cellular distribution in the GCA arteries is as follows: (1) immune cells: dendritic cells, T cells, monocytes, macrophages, and to a lower extent B cells (2) vascular cells: endothelial cells and vascular smooth muscle cells [11]. GCA artery

TLR fingerprint consist of high amounts of TLR2, TLR4 and TLR8, intermediate levels of the TLR1, TLR5, and TLR6 and lower or absent for TLR3 and TLR9 [11]. TLRs of vascular DCs are implicated in the strong tissue tropism of GCA [11].

In GCA, most severe inflammatory effects occur at the intima/media border, adjacent to the internal elastic lamina from the outside in, from the adventitia to the intima direction [14], but sometimes the inflammation is initiated in a tiny area in the vasa vasorum in intra-adventitial small vessels [31].

2.1.2 Recruitment, proliferation, and polarization of T cells into GCA arteries

Already activated adventitial DCs produce cytokines and chemokines (C-C motif chemokine ligand) CCL 19, 20, and 21 that trigger the recruitment of CD4+ T cell subpopulation, in proximity to vascular DCs [4, 36]. They in turn proliferate and synthesize chemokines (including CD4, CD61), creating an inflammatory environment [12]. Under the influence of the DCs and modulated by immune checkpoints [36], CD 4+ T cells subpopulation [37] differentiate into T helper 1 (Th1) cells and T helper 17 (Th 17) cells [38]. Next, T cells polarize into two T cell lineages defined by the production of their marker cytokines Th1 cells start producing interferon gamma (IFN_γ), while Th17 cells produce interleukins IL17 and IL21 [38]. IFNv-releasing T cells axis and IL17/21 T cells axis, respectively, have different immunomodulatory effects [4].

IL-12 and IL 23 stimulate Th1 and Th17 responses, respectively, both of which are believed to be involved in promoting systemic and vascular inflammation, progression, and maintenance of inflammation [39, 40].

Interleukin 6 is the cytokine that controls the balance between proinflammatory Th1 and Th17 cells and the regulatory T cells, particularly involved in GCA pathogenesis [4, 41]. Regulatory T cells normally ponder or inhibit the immune system response. The disturbance of T cell homeostasis is probably related to an imbalance in the amount of serum IL6 [42]. In patients with GCA, IL 6 is upregulated in the inflamed arteries and in circulation [5, 42]. Serum IL6 corelates with disease activity and is decreased when GCA is in remission [42]. T proinflammatory cells Th1 and Th17 are in excess [38], while regulatory T cell numbers are inhibited by excess interleukin 6 (IL 6) [42].

Upon T cell activation in presence of an antiself attack [14], inhibitory checkpoints such as T-cell–inducible immune checkpoint programmed death-1/programmed death ligand-1 (PD-1/PD-L1) pathway are instrumental to minimize potential immunopathology [36]. PD1/PD-L1 pathway has a role in maintenance of tolerance, protective immunity, preventing autoimmunity disease, and protection against collateral vascular damage [36]. PD-1 is expressed on activated T and DCs cells [36] and its coupling by its ligands PD-L1 or PD-L2 induces T cell receptor (TCR)-activation cascade in a Src homology region 2 domain-containing phosphatase 2 (SHP2) manner [36], resulting in immunosuppression. An aberrant PD-1/PD-L1 checkpoint in DCs (low amount of both PD1/PDL1) and T cells of GCA patients [36] is responsible for the observed DC-mediated hyperactivation of T cells, polarizing T cells to Th1 and Th17 [36]. The immunotolerance defect in regulatory T cells in GCA patients [41] is characterized by a stimulatory instead of inhibitory function of PD1-mediated immune checkpoint in GCA patients [36], followed downstream by a FOXP3 transcription factor defect in the regulatory T cells locally in GCA arterial lesions [41] which leads to decrease in the number of FoxP3+ T regulatory cells and hyperstimulation of proinflammatory T cells. In addition, the regulatory T cell population can be influenced with an IL6 receptor antagonist [41] which stresses the necessity of IL6 in these processes. Importantly, IL17 is controlled rapidly by glucocorticoids [4]. IFNy is resistant to corticoids, also to aspirin and NOTCH inhibitors [4, 43].

2.1.3 Monocytes differentiation/macrophages role in GCA-related vascular damage

Under an increased level of interferon-gamma (IFNγ) produced by CD+4 T cells, monocytes and macrophages are recruited in the arterial wall [44]. IFNv primarily targets macrophages leading to their fusion together into giant cells (GC) [4, 44]. IFNv concentration was found to be elevated in arterial tissue from GCA patients with ischemic disturbances, including visual loss [44]. In addition, they reported patients with PMR and fever had elevated IL2 production [44].

Using *ex vivo* cultures of temporal artery biopsies, Cid et al., 2006 demonstrated that the role of IFNy is to induce the production of C-C motif chemokine ligand 2 (CCL2) (ligand of CCR2 receptor) by VSMCs [45, 46]. CCR2, the corresponding receptor, is also expressed by monocytes, binding of CCR2 on monocytes leads to the recruitment of monocytes and their differentiation inside all layers of the arterial wall [46]. INFy induces the production of C-X-C motif chemokine ligand (CXCL9, 10, 11) by VSMCs [46], linked to the recruitment of cells expressing CXCR3 which is expressed by Th1 cells and CD8+ cells [4]. This will initiate a positive feedback loop since T cells are being activated and produce more IFNy [4, 46, 47].

Macrophages have different functions depending on which vascular layer they are going to be trapped in (1) adventitial CD 68+ TGF β1+ macrophages produce proinflammatory cytokines IL1β and IL 6 [4, 11, 48]; (2) intimal-media junction macrophages secrete metalloproteinases to clear cellular debris. They are also responsible for unintended, pathological elastic membranes digestion; (3) macrophages in the intima layer have roles in cellular outgrowth [49]. Intima-located macrophages led to production platelet-derived growth factor (PDGF) [50] which is needed for dedifferentiation, proliferation and migration of VSMCs [50, 51] and vascular endothelial growth factor (VEGF) which is needed for neoangiogenesis [52].

IL1β and IL 6 levels are influenced by GS in GCA [43], in contrast, IL12 is mostly resistant to GS therapy [4, 18]. The lack of reaction to GS suggests a need for better therapeutic strategies to interfere with these pathologic cascades.

Monocytes and macrophages accumulate in high numbers generating granulomatous inflammation of large and medium arteries and, under stimulatory influence of INFv, they form giant cells (GC) by fusing together [4, 5].

In physiological conditions, GC are the body defense response against a foreign body or a kind of irritant, for instance, a splinter in the finger, the body will produce GCs to break up this irritant and remove it. In the case of GCA, 'the foreign body' is not known. It has been stated by some authors that it might be the arteriosclerotic plaque [53]. Macrophage multinucleated giant cells in pathological conditions of GCA are a unique cell population that produce different mediators leading to the destruction and faulty reconstruction of the arterial wall [4, 54].

3. Vascular remodeling of healthy arteries to GCA arteries

Regarding the GCA pathophysiology, studies have observed many interchangeable features dictated by the 'confused' immune system and by the cellular populations of the vascular wall itself mediated by blood factors. Upon the destructive actions of GCs, the vessel initiates a faulty PDGF- [50] and VEGF- [55] dependent maladaptive reparatory mechanism [55].

GCs' proteases digest the vascular wall at the level of the internal elastic lamina [54, 56, 57]. For instance, media-intima junction GCs are producing metalloproteinases (MMP-9 and MMP2) [57] as was demonstrated recently [54, 57], and also other mediators. VEGF [55] is linked to neoangiogenesis and the recruitment of proinflammatory T cells via Notch/Jagged 1 dependent pathway [4, 5], reactive oxygen species (ROS) [54], and the other inflammatory mediators with proteolytic activity that cause breakage of the internal elastic lamina. The vascular response is a result of the two-way interaction between the hyperactive immune cells and the activated vascular cells. These processes lead to: (1) release of additional growth factors; (2) release of vWF from ECs Weibel-Palade bodies [19, 58–61]; (3) release of macrophage factors [13, 44, 48]; (4) media thickening in response to the immune insult [50] and deposition of extracellular matrix proteins (i.e. collagen); (5) intima myofibrotic hyperplasia (IH) [50]; (6) release of angiogenic factors in the vasa vasorum [62]; and finally, (7) upregulation of the proteinases [54] and downregulation of their inhibitors which causes the intima elastic membrane to tear [54], destroying locally the vessel wall.

Most importantly, the increased production of such mediators as PDGF [50, 51] and endothelin-1 [63, 64], initiates a faulty vascular repair process, leading to the activation, dedifferentiation, proliferation, and migration of the VSMCs from the arterial media to the intima. This leads to myofibrous intimal hyperplasia and "nodular" media thickening with granulomatous giant multinucleated cells infiltration, and neoangiogenic vasa vasorum [44, 62] characteristic to GCA pathology [51]. Typically, VSMCs turn from a contractile cell into a dedifferentiated, secretory, and migratory cell [5, 65]. Activated and injured vascular smooth muscle cells (VSMCs) produce growth factors (including PDGFs [55], TGF-β and ET-1 [63, 64]) that promote further myofibroblast dedifferentiation, proliferation and migration [4]. Reversely, pharmacologic blockage of the PDGF receptor or blockage ET-1 receptors [64] results in reduced IH in cultured GCA arteries [51, 64].

In all, hyperplastic cell outgrowth in the lumen of medium sized artery through autoimmune vascular remodeling progressively narrows the lumen, resulting in vascular stenosis and ischemia in the distal organs these vessels normally irrigate. The eye and the brain are at highest risk. The invalidating or life-threating consequences are severe, possibly visual loss or even stroke. Patients with GCA who have ocular ischemic complications have higher blood concentrations of ET-1 and other EC biomarkers, highlighting these biomarker potential role in thromboembolic vascular disturbances [63, 64].

3.1 The crosstalk between immune cells/vascular cells, faulty vascular repair and thrombosis in primary vasculitis

More and more evidence suggests the presence of crosstalk between mispositioned vascular inflammation [4] and thrombosis [5, 61, 66]. In the past the underlying molecular mechanisms of vasculitis have been overlooked, but more recently, it has become increasingly evident that inflammatory diseases of the blood vessels are associated with arterial [25, 67] and venous thrombosis [66]. In GCA, certain risk factors will seriously increase the likeliness of thrombotic events, including, but not limited to systemic inflammation, localized vascular inflammation, endothelial dysfunction and treatment-related complications [5, 68]. The higher risk of thrombosis during active disease underlines the role of inflammation in thrombogenesis [61, 68]. Furthermore, GCA patients have a greater risk of thromboembolic complications due to the advanced age, and to the other risk factors that they concomitantly have, such as hypertension, smoking, hypercholesterolemia, previous arterial thrombotic events, family history of thrombosis, and the presence of additional cardiovascular risk factors [25, 28, 61, 68]. This may contribute to the choice of administrating antithrombotic therapy: low dose aspirin 75–250 milligram per day prevents cerebrovascular events and ocular symptoms [69]. Antiplatelet therapy influences arterial disease events [69], while anticoagulants and immunosuppressive medication have a debatable effect [21, 70].

3.1.1 Immune cells response in vasculitis

A growing body of evidence supports the above-mentioned 'outside-in' hypothesis that vascular inflammation is initiated and perpetuated in the adventitia in GCA and contributes progressively to medial and intimal remodeling [14]. Once the immune barrier is broken [12], the vessel expresses cell surface adhesion molecules in the vasa vasorum [55] and inflammatory mediators [5]. In result, the monocytes migrate towards the intima of the blood vessels [53]. Th1 and Th17 T-cells pathogenic pathways promote the production of IFN-y and, respectively IL-17 [38, 38]. Th17 differentiation via its effector IL17 pathways induce chronic inflammation [71]. B cell differentiation contribute less to the formation of granulomatous structures [4, 5]. Cytokines like TNF alpha, interleukins IL1β and IL6 are promoting not only systemic signs in primary vasculitis (fever, malaise, weight loss, fatigue) but they also favor a prothromboembolic state [61, 67]. GCA complications comprise arterial [67] and, although less frequent, venous involvement, both DVT and PE [66]. In mouse models of DVT, it has been demonstrated high IL 6 during thrombogenesis [72], while inhibition of IL6 reduces expression of CCL2 which leads to a low recruitment of monocytes at the site of thrombosis of the vessel wall and the post-thrombotic syndrome [72]. IL6 is triggering an amplification and recruitment of monocytes which is in relation to the ability to express in excess cell adhesion molecules in vasa vasorum [4]. One puzzling observation from published data is that IL 6 pleiotropic effects on immune and vascular cells assert disease activity in GCA, however, when IL6 expression in the temporal artery is low, the IL6-induced angiogenic response is decreased without a protection mechanism against ischemic events in GCA patient [42]. Acute phase proteins are elevated: serum amyloid A (SAA), CRP, ESR, WBC count and platelet count [1]. GCA patients having ocular complications have significantly decreased level of SAA, CRP and ESR [27] as well as high VCAM1 levels [73]. GCA patients during relapses had significantly higher levels of SAA, CRP, ESR and WBC counts [73, 74].

Hyperactivated T cells and macrophages organize the granulomatous lesions in the vessel wall [44], destroy the media layer, the inflamed artery initiates an abnormal vascular repair program [11], inducing ischemic organ damage through intimal hyperplasia and luminal occlusion changes [5, 36]. Elevated IFNv was demonstrated to be correlated with neoangiogenesis [4, 62], and IH [46], two critical processes in vascular remodeling in GCA artery. Persistence of IFNv correlates with chronical arterial inflammatory disease [4]. Clinical variations in GCA are correlated with local expression of cytokine mRNA (elevated IL1β, IL6, TGF, IL2, INFy, IL17, 13). Heterogeneity of immune response and targeting of the arterial tissue in a TLR-specific manner explain the diverse clinical manifestations inside GCA spectrum of diseases [4, 11].

3.1.2 Vascular wall response to vasculitis

In GCA pathogenesis it is thought that the vascular wall response has the same impact as the immune cell response [4].

3.1.2.1 Arterial luminal vs. vasa vasorum endothelial cells response in GCA

Vascular endothelial dysfunction was previously reported in GCA [53]. It is associated with elevated blood levels of proinflammatory endothelial factors that have important roles in the pathogenesis of GCA: endothelin 1 (ET-1, [64]), and cell adhesion molecules [19, 64, 75], and von Willebrand factor (VWF) [19, 20, 53, 59]. The presence of the proinflammatory and procoagulant factors at GCA lesions sites is indicative of the extensive crosstalk between immune system and vascular cells [61]. The contribution of the blood vessel wall to the GCA pathogenesis is stressed by the fact that symmetrical, collateral vessels are much more likely to be affected (implicating GCA strong tissue tropism [4] in contrast to, for instance, atherosclerotic diffuse display which also manifests in this age group [53]) as demonstrated in these patients by PET scans/CT angiography imaging [17, 73].

Thrombin, the main protease in the coagulation cascade, also has numerous effects on the endothelium, i.e. thrombin-induced expression of chemokines that trigger binding of platelets and monocytes to the endothelial surface [76] and increased permeability across endothelium [77]. By these and many other mechanisms [78], thrombin is coupling coagulation and inflammation [61, 78, 79]. The stimulatory effects of thrombin on ECs and platelets occur mainly through activation of the protease-activated receptors (PARs) [79]. PARs are seven-trans-membrane G protein coupled signaling proteins [80]. PAR1 is the prototype for a family of four related receptors [79]. PAR1 is the key mediator of thrombin's effect on human ECS [79]. Thrombin activates PAR1 receptors which couple to $G\alpha q/11$ and $G\alpha 12/13$ that upregulate the vWF and P-selectin secretion from the ECs storage granules named Weibel Palade bodies (WPBs) [79, 81, 82]. Soluble P-selectin is an adhesive molecule also stored in WPBs [81]. Relevantly, P-selectin secreted by luminal endothelium of the carotid artery in a murine vascular damage model was reported to be involved in monocyte trafficking and neointima formation [65].

One of the mechanisms that may cause endothelial dysfunction in primary vasculitis is the excess of proinflammatory cytokines that are depressing endothelial function [31]. Also, the inflammatory microenvironment is directly leading t0 endothelial cell toxicity. In addition, healthy and pathological damaged cells are intercommunicating and interconnecting, for instance monocytes and GC interactions close to the vessel wall trigger endothelial damage. Another role of the endothelium in inflammation is in leukocyte trafficking (P-selectin, E-selectins expression) [55] and the expression of cell adhesion molecules in the vasa vasorum [55]. Transcript levels for markers of endothelial activation: VWF, ICAM1, VCAM1, CD31, VE-cadherin (and of myofibroblasts smooth muscle cells actin (SMA)) measured by RT-PCR in the tissues in a GCA mouse model [36] were found to be elevated by up to fourfold when PD-1 was blocked with anti-PD-1 Ab when compared with control IgG or vehicle-treated [36] immune checkpoint inhibition led to intimal hyperplasia, angiogenesis and nodular thickening of the media. Inflammation-induced effects caused by the endothelium in systemic inflammation disease include but are not limited to: (1) increased expression of procoagulant factors: VWF, plasminogen activator inhibitor 1 (PAI1), platelets activated factor (PAF), vascular cell adhesion molecule 1 (VCAM1), intercellular adhesion molecule (ICAM1) and tissue factor (TF) and (2) and inhibition of anticoagulation pathways and fibrinolysis activity: endothelial protein C receptor (EPCR), tissue plasminogen activator (tPA), thrombomodulin (TM), prostaglandin I 2 (PGI2), that are causing thrombotic tendency [61, 83]. In patients with visual disturbances there were reported high VCAM1 levels compared with GCA patients that did not have visual disturbances [73]. VCAM1 was also significantly correlated with large vessel envolvement [73].

Weibel-Palade bodies (WPBs) are the secretory granules of vascular ECs [81]. The main resident of WPBs is vWF [81, 84]. vWF is pro-inflammatory and pro-thrombotic agent which plays a central role in morbidity and mortality associated with systemic inflammation and cardiovascular disease. The fact that elevated vWF in the circulation is a marker of inflammation-induced activation of ECs is well established [82, 85], but why do activated endothelial cell release von Willebrand factor in the context of the pro-inflammatory microenvironment in vasculitis, in particular in GCA, by which mechanism, is not completely understood; it was suggested it is part of the reparatory process. When an immune checkpoint is inhibited, endothelial cells are bigger in size and increased VWF expression and secretion was reported [36], indicative of endothelial cell maladaptive reaction. Moreover, VEGF derived from macrophages and the other immune cells have a stimulatory influence on Weibel-Palade bodies' secretion of VWF and angiopoetin-2 [86] involved in neointima formation. Intriguingly, it was reported that PDGF released by vascular dendritic cells [55] -on top of the above-described proinflammatory features- regulates vWF gene promoter.

vWF is an important molecular link coupling thrombosis and inflammation. It was found to contribute to systemic and vascular inflammatory manifestations of GCA. VWF levels are elevated in GCA patients circulation up to three-folds [19]. Highest vWF values are recorded at the onset of the disease [19], high blood VWF levels are persistent throughout the active disease period and remain elevated in some patients a long time after corticosteroid treatment [19, 59]. According to Persellin et al. elevated blood vWF values are not due to impairment of vWF formation or storage but to increased ECs secretion of normal von Willebrand factor, as shown by electrophoretic analysis of high molecular weight vWF polymers pattern [20]. High active VWF levels reflect vascular distress that predicts the course of the disease towards vasoocclusive problems [20]. Intraluminal thromboses were seen in 10% in TAB+ GCA, but in fact, the rate might be higher and hidden by the concomitant hyperplastic reaction in the intima. Several studies proposed VWF could be a parameter to monitor treatment or a parameter for diagnosis when the acute phase reactants (ESR) are normal in treated GCA patients. The fact that elevation of VWF is persistent throughout the steroid treatment suggests that GS treatment has little effect on the underlying endothelial disease. A significant percentage of patients receiving steroid treatment are developing irreversible vascular occlusive complications episodes (%) even after receiving GS treatment [67].

Several studies investigated the role of vWF in the formation of the hyperplasic intima (IH) [58, 60]. In one study, matching TABs and matching blood collection was done for VWF measurement. Increased vWF deposition in hyperplastic neointima mirrored high plasma vWF levels [19]. These data and other published data- that increased levels of vWF are associated with hyperplasia in grafts [87], and no occurrence of atherosclerotic plaques in vWF deficient pigs [88] -suggests a role for vWF in vascular remodeling and faulty vacular repair [60, 75]. Indeed, in a recent study by Lagrange et al. [58] it was found that vWF/LRP4/integrin α vβ3 axis stimulates proliferation of VSMCs: (1) vWF binds through its A2 domain to the VSMCs LRP4 receptor; (2) crosstalk LRP4 receptor-integrin α vβ3; (3) integrin α vβ3 activates Src signaling leading to vWF-dependent VSMCs proliferation [58]. Relevant to the aim of this review, their new findings provide new insights into the pathogenic mechanisms that drive pathological hyperplasia of the GCA arterial vessel wall. Moreover, the vWF/LRP4/integrin α vβ3 axis may represent a novel therapeutic target to inhibit VSMC proliferation, and, at least partially, prevent the maladaptive reparatory process in GCA [58].

At high shear-rates-which is the case in our pathogenetic context in the artery stenosis provoked by vascular remodeling in select ischemic complications of GCA, the inactive, globular circulating vWF unfolds into a highly active HMW elongated conformation. The active, elongated vWF can bind platelets via its repetitive A1 domain forming'beads on a string' conformations the incipient steps of thrombus formation [82]. von Willebrand factor, then, has a two-way pathogenic mechanism to actively participate in GCA artery occlusion, on one hand, because at the site of the autoimmune vascular lesion, VWF, released from systemic inflammation thrombin-activated vascular ECs, initiates platelet adhesion, and changes the thrombotic propensity [19, 59], and on the other hand, amplifies maladaptive vascular response via vWF/integrin axis [58], based on these published data it is highly probably that the rate of intraluminal thrombotic events is higher than expected and the rate of TIA in GCA patients is also probably to be higher. It is worth mentioning here that episodes of transient visual loss precede permanent visual loss in 44% of cases [27]. To conclude, these two roles of vWF in GCA arteries are most likely associated with poor outcome of cerebral, coronary, or ocular ischemic complications of GCA disease [67]; leading in some people to type 2 GCA-related myocardial infarction [25, 26]. The highest VWF levels were recorded in GCA patients with positive temporal arteries biopsy when associating ocular symptoms [20], further studies are needed for vWF role in the ischemic complications of GCA. Reversely, in PMR, they reported lower levels of VWF than in GCA, which might be indicative of a lower degree of endothelial dysfunction, in PMR it correlates with the severity of the clinical signs, "more fuel on the fire" in the course of the disease [20]. For all these purposes, accurate criteria for active GCA disease are needed.

GCA relapsing cases or cases unresponsive to corticosteroid therapy that also have high blood VWF levels, high ESR, eye symptoms, would be candidates for testing new prospective therapeutics that either block vWF release from ECs activated by inflammatory cytokines in GCA [19] or block the mitogenic effect of vWF on IH [58].

3.1.2.2 Vasa vasorum ECs response to vasculitis

In response to activated vascular DCs in the adventitial layer, the invasion of multiple types of immune cells is currently thought to occur through the vasa vasorum endothelium [4]. The question to ask is why and how endothelial cells of the tiny adventitial vessels allow the immune cells to break into the vascular wall of the GCA arteries. The role of vasa vasorum ECs is major in GCA pathogenesis though the molecular details are still cryptic. In PMR and GCA as well, adventitial macrophages stimulated by DCs produce IL6 and IL1 which are detected from the early stages, when temporal artery is histologically apparent normal and the INFy expressing T cells are still absent from the vascular wall [11, 13]. At these early stages it is expected that vasa vasorum ECs are activated, express selectins and have a role in increasing wall permeability. In the same time, new vasa vasorum are formed, not only in the adventitia, but across all layers of arterial wall. Their role is to transport the invading immune cells.

3.1.3 Platelets response to vascular inflammation

Platelets are activated by the following activated EC factors: (1) increased thromboxane A2; (2) increased von Willebrand factor and (3) decreased prostaglandin I2 [83]. Platelets are activated by the pro-inflammatory cytokines expressed by ECs and immune cells, by PAF, and by thrombin [83]. When activated, platelets secrete P-selectin and directly interact with endothelial cells [83]. Activated platelets interact with monocytes and neutrophils through the NF-KB mediated pathway [4, 83]. Activated platelets release pro-inflammatory cytokines or chemokines (like IL1 and CD 40) [4, 83]. Activated platelets are involved in microparticle-mediated inflammation [83].

3.2 Thromboembolic complications in GCA patients-clinical features and pathophysiological data subsidiary to vascular dysfunction

3.2.1 Arterial thrombotic complications in GCA

Most common clinical features in GCA patients are the ischemic symptoms: headache, jaw claudication and visual symptoms. If not promptly treated, GCA can lead to systemic complications: aortic aneurysm and rupture, and to ischemic complications of GCA: myocardial infarction, stroke, and blindness. Patients with GCA are experiencing these syndromes due the progressive vessel stenosis/occlusion of the affected arteries, secondary to vascular damage and IH. Several pathogenic mechanisms could explain the increased risk of thromboembolic complications in patients with GCA, including immune and vascular cell aging [89], stasis, endothelial dysfunction, hypercoagulability, and decreased fibrinolysis, the features of inflammatory-derived thrombosis.

3.2.1.1 Cranial symptoms-involvement of intra carotid artery and vertebrobasilar branches

Cranial symptoms are classically associated with GCA: new onset headaches, the most common initial symptom, typical in temporal area but can be diffuse/nonspecific, persistent throughout the day, partly responsive to analgesics; scalp tenderness seen in 50% of patients; usually noticed while brushing hair; temporal artery abnormalities pulse; jaw claudication is seen in 50% of patients, the most specific symptom of arteritis, is a mandibular pain brought on by speech and mastication, relieved when stopping the activities, highly suggestive of GCA, strongly associated with positive TAB. In rare cases, muscles of the tongue and swallowing may be affected.

3.2.1.2 Stroke in GCA

Most strokes in the investigated GCA patients were found in the vertebrobasilar and internal carotid artery territory [33, 90]. The reported rate of stroke/transient ischemic attack (TIA) is approximately 5–20% [25, 33]. The underlying mechanism of cerebrovascular ischemia is related to the vascular dysfunction that is characteristic of GCA. More recent GCA studies [28, 33, 67] reported a 2.8% -7% incidence of ischemic stroke. As mentioned on previous section, a lot of inflammatory cells collect around internal elastic lamina but intracranial arteries lack an internal elastic lamina that being one of the reasons stroke is not seen as a severe manifestation of GCA in that territory.

In a cohort study evaluating the thrombotic risk in GCA patients vs. control it was found an increased risk of cerebrovascular accidents like in the other studies, and also peripheric arteritis and myocardial infarction [25]. The incidence rate ratio for CV events was 1.68 [25]. There is a significantly increased risk of thromboembolic disease in GCA during active disease; the risk for thrombotic events was reportedly the highest in the first month from the onset of the disease hazard ratio 4.92 (95% CI 2.59–9.34. The risk for CV risk was much decreased at a follow-up (hazard ratio of 1.70) (95% CI 1.51–1.91) [25]. Although patients with GCA have an increased risk of cerebrovascular accidents, long-term survival study concluded that GCA patients' mortality is not higher than in the general population if treated properly [34].

3.2.1.3 Visual symptoms-internal carotid artery branches involvement

Blindness is the most severe thromboembolic event experienced by 15–20% of GCA patients, usually at onset [6, 27]. It is rarely reversible. Visual loss is abrupt and painless and the most feared consequence of GCA by the clinicians. GCA is an ophthalmology emergency which requires 'emergency' IV pulse therapy with high dose prednisolone followed by oral therapy to prevent progression in the affected eye and extension to the contralateral eye [21].

Transient monocular visual loss (TMVL) or amaurosis fugax means a person cannot see through one or both eyes, a symptom of poor blood supply to the eye(s). TMVL is seen in 10–15% of patients. If left untreated 50% of cases are rapidly progressing to permanent visual loss (VL). Unilateral VL is a strong risk factor for VL in the contralateral eye which can occur in more than 50% of cases within 2 weeks if left untreated [27].

VL is usually due to arteritic anterior ischemic optic neuropathy: occlusive arteritis of the posterior ciliary branches of the ophthalmic artery which are the main arterial supply of the optic nerve [91]; it accounts for 85% of all VL cases in GCA [27, 91]. VL can also be due to central retinal artery occlusion or posterior ischemic optic neuropathy [27, 33, 91]. Other ocular symptoms in GCA might be ophthalmoplegia and diplopia from ischemia of the extraocular muscles and blurry vision [27].

Intriguingly, one of the acute phase reactants, an innate immunity pattern recognition receptor, pentraxin 3(PTX3) accumulates at the site of active vascular remodeling, more so in GCA patients with recent ocular ischemic events ischemia [52], indicative of thrombo-inflammation manifestations in GCA vessels that supply the eye, as shown by immunohistochemistry and measurement of plasma levels of PTX3 [52].

3.2.1.4 Extracranial/large vessel involvement

Extracranial/large vessel involvement refers to involvement of aorta and its major branch vessels. About 25–30% of GCA cases have clinically evident large vessel involvement [90] but PET scans and CT angiography have demonstrated that subclinical large vessel involvement is present in a significant percentage of cases [90]. The GCA vasculopathy may evolve to aneurysm formation and vascular rupture of aorta and stenosis/occlusion of its branch vessels [68]. Clinically, these patients may present extremity claudication, absent peripheral pulses, abdominal pain, masked HTA, dizziness depending on affected vessels. Because of risk of vascular stenosis, it is needed an evaluation of the blood supply. If decreased blood supply is found, the question is if this is part of GCA occlusive complications or related to artherosclerosis which is almost universal in people in this age group that develop GCA or both. Leg vessels are less involved in GCA than the arm, the neck, the brain, or the eye vessels, but vascular complications can occur in the leg too, just less frequently. Blood pressure and pulses discrepancies of 15-20 mg between left and right extremities might raises question of large vessel arteritis involvement and might hide hypertension.

3.2.2 Venous thrombotic complications in GCA

In a cohort study of circa one thousand GCA patients, an increased risk of venous thromboembolism was observed (both DVT and pulmonary embolism), during the early active, uncontrolled phase of the disease [66].

Nevertheless, with appropriate health care, giant cell arteritis has a relatively good prognosis.

4. Vascular remodeling is the 'unmet need' in GCA treatment-standard therapy and future perspectives

4.1 Glucocorticosteroids treatment-advantages and disadvantages

The glucocorticosteroids (GS) remain the drug of choice for the GCA treatment. In presence of the characteristic clinical signs, GCA is diagnosed by using the Westergren method, high erythrocyte precipitate is indicative of this inflammatory condition and the indication is to start the GS therapy without delay and followed up with a biopsy of the temporal artery [29]. GS treatment is started with about 1 mg/kg/day prednisone and then is tapered at 3, 6, 9 and 12 months-a long taper with intend to withdraw GS around 12–24 months [29]. GCA disease, if treated properly, has an excellent prognosis, but it is difficult for most people to be tapered off prednisone entirely. Most GCA patients must take low dose prednisone daily for months and years. GCA patients are elderly people, a prednisone hit on top of a frail constitution leads to higher disease toll compared to if the disease would occur earlier in life.

About 50% patient relapse after a mean follow up of 7 months at a mean prednisone dose of 4 mg/day [29]. Furthermore, GS are generating side effects, about 90% of patients receiving prednisone for GCA will have at least one GCA-related side effect after 1 year [29].

The question to ask is what we can add or substitute for GS to get tide control of the disease and address the unmet need of vascular luminal changes. GS are easing the symptoms quickly, by blocking inflammatory responses, probably correlated with the rapid decrease in the serum IL 6 and blockage of activation, proliferation, and polarization of the T cells, in particular of Th17 cells. Therefore, GS are still the best available treatment for the induction and remission of GCA, but, unfortunately, they fail to resorb the vessel wall infiltrates or to attenuate the underlying vascular dysfunction pathogenic mechanisms. It is not well known how GS intervene on systemic inflammation's vascular component in GCA, but for instance Cid et al. 2000 reported that GS treatment was not sufficient to completely abrogate the expression of adhesion molecules, [55] in their patients, indicating a persistent exposure of ECs and VSMCs cells to a remaining inflammatory microenvironment despite the rapid symptomatic improvement achieved at follow-up after GS treatment. Moreover, GS have no effect on the restoration of regulatory T cells, and mild effect on TH1 polarization [21, 29]. Another interesting study on 40 patients with TAB+ GCA treated with prednisone, in which they had a randomization for follow-up TABs at 3, 6, 9 and 12 months, has shown that in 50% of cases, positive TAB histopathologic signs were still present after one year of GS treatment, showing GS have little to zero effect on vascular remodeling [21, 92, 93]. Vascular remodeling remains the unmet need of current GCA therapy [43, 93]. Therefore, it is very important to develop new strategies to spare GS in GCA. Some of the drugs proposed in the past are toxic or ineffective [5].

The other drug that is recommended for almost all GCA patients is low dose aspirin (85 mg a day) because it decreases the risk of developing subsequential visual loss or cerebrovascular events in giant cell arteritis [69], and it addresses any thrombogenic tendency in blood vessels supplying the eye and the CNS. Some more recent studies challenge the benefit of using aspirin in GCA treatment [5]. The use of otherconventional anticoagulant therapy for the thromboembolic complications of GCA remains controversial and is not recommended [5, 70].

Up to more recent date, the only GS-saving agent was methotrexate [5]. It was demonstrated in a metanalysis gathering phase III randomized blind controlled trials on 161 patients that methotrexate decreases the risk of GCA relapses and is able of GS-saving effect [43].

4.2 Experimental models of GCA

In most to-date published studies, the biochemical assays were conducted on cultured human arteries collected by TAB from GCA patients compared with healthy cultured arterial cells, according to protocol from healthy subjects unrelated to GCA and on peripheral blood collected from GCA patients.

Several murine models of large vessel vasculitis are currently available [5, 43]. Some murine models are KO for genes which encode proteins that have crucial roles in GCA pathogenesis. IL1 rn−/− mice are lacking the gene encoding for the IL 1 receptor antagonist and it was found that these mice develop T-cell dependent vasculitis [5, 43]. Others used herpes virus-infected mouse models of vasculitis [10]. Another model involved microsurgery and physical contact of the murine aorta with an elastase to destroy the vascular wall and mice developed aortitis [5, 43].

The most interesting systemic murine model developed by Weyand group [4] uses implant of human temporal artery (allowing dissection of specific GCA pathogenetic mechanisms) or infusion of human peripheral blood monocytes from GCA patients in severely immunodeficient mice [38]. The model of subcutaneous engraftment of human TAB+ GCA arteries in severely immunodeficient mice opened the possibility to test new biologics therapy effects on immune cells and its afferent GCA artery, both cells and GCA artery originating from the specific patient in the murine model of GCA, maybe allowing in future studies collection of predictive data on how a specific GCA patient would react to the administrated drug of choice [4].

4.3 GS-sparing agents for GCA treatment

4.3.1 Tocilizumab and GiACTA study

One of the most important therapeutic targets for the treatment of GCA disease is related to IL6.

Tocilizumab is a monoclonal antibody targeted against IL6 receptor α [94]. IL6 is the cytokine that controls the balance between regulatory T cells, Th17 and Th1 which is particularly involved in GCA pathogenesis. Collectively, IL6 published data leaded to the breakthrough Giant cell Arteritis Actemra (GiACTA) study was published in 2017 by Stone et al. [94]. GiACTA is a global, randomized, double blind, double placebo-controlled Phase III trial evaluating efficacy and safety of tocilizumab in active GCA in which there were compared 4 groups: in two groups people where receiving IL6 receptor antagonist tocilizumab every week or every other week in association with prednisone over 6 months or 1 year; in the two placebo groups patients were receiving prednisone either 6 months or 1 year [94]. The primary outcome measurement at one year was the sustained remission (56% of the patients in weekly tocilizumab group and 53% in those receiving every other week tocilizumab group compared to only 14% in the short-course prednisone without tocilizumab group, of a total of 251 patients) [95]. GiACTA results demonstrates the superiority of tocilizumab to placebo non-dependent on the duration of prednisone, sustained remission, excluding CRP concentration normalization [94].

GiACTA lead to the FDA approval of tocilizumab in 2017 as first and only specific therapy to treat GCA in the USA and Europe [30, 95], in combination with protocol-defined dose of GS. Tocilizumab successful clinical trials indicate that blockage of IL-6-dependent inflammatory pathways strongly inhibits systemic inflammation as well as PMR and ocular syndrome in GCA patients [30, 95]. Tocilizumab prescription is particularly useful in corticodependance and severe adverse reactions to GS (osteoporosis, diabetics, HTA) [30, 95].

There were a few reports of what happens after tocilizumab withdrawal. In an effort to optimize the tocilizumab treatment duration, a multicenter prospective open label study investigated the risk of relapse associated with tocilizumab discontinuation after new GCA patients received 4 infusions of tocilizumab at weeks 0, 4, 8 and 12 wks [5, 43]. They observed that this treatment can be very effective, but after tocilizumab termination, at least in some patients (25%), it was seen relapse revival [43]. Same, in a long-term follow-up of the GiACTA study confirmed on larger number of patients, in which the treatment was stopped at one year, the relapse revival decrease was seen and it was more comparable between groups after two years follow-up [43, 93]. Importantly, there is no proof of tocilizumab efficacy on vascular remodeling. One of the molecular effects of IL-6 blockade was reported by Terrades-Garcia et al. who investigated the molecular effects of tocilizumab; for this study temporal arteries from 13 GCA patients and 8 controls were cultured with or without tocilizumab. After 5 days of culture, tocilizumab selectively induced a decrease in CXC 13 chemokine mRNA expression in cultured arteries, and they concluded disruption of B cell homeostasis may partially account for the therapeutic effects of tocilizumab (ACR meeting 2016), with no significant changes in other chemokines [5]. Further studies are needed to identify predictive factors of relapses.

4.3.2 Therapeutical targets-updates and controversies

METOGia is a currently conducted, randomized controlled clinical study comparing administration tocilizumab for one year with one-year treatment of methotrexate in association with protocol-controlled prednisone [43].

A new IL1R antagonist (anakinra) effects in GCA treatment is currently under clinical trial, with promising perspective [43].

Activated T cells could be moderated by inference at immunoinhibitory checkpoints [36]. A potential drug intervention is to control excessive TH cell activation and invasion along arterial wall by using abatacerpt. Abatacept is a recombinant fusion protein made from fragment of human Ig1 fused to a domain of cytotoxic T-lymphocyte-associated antigen 4 (which is usually expressed on stimulated T cells) used in vasculitis with positive results, mild efficacy [96], mild GC-sparing effect [5]. There is an ongoing Phase III clinical trial [93].

Blocking IL-12/23 by binding to their common p40 subunit, with another monoclonal antibody ustekinumab has according to one report a positive influence in relapsing GCA [97]. Ustekinumab administered after rapid decrease in GS dose did not prevent disease relapse in one recent small study [98], it still has an open trial label for comparative multicenter study comparing GS alone treatment to GS and ustekinumab in refractory GCA [43].

Macrophages' activation various pathways (mediated by IFN-y, TNFα, CSF-2/ CSF-2R (CSF-2: colony-stimulating factor 2), IL 6/IL-6 receptor) [2] should be therapeutically targeted in GCA to prevent blood vessel destruction [54, 56] and the faulty vascular reparatory remodeling [2, 38, 54, 57, 62]. For instance, mavrilimumab is another agent under clinical trial for GCA treatment, targeting macrophage CSF-2/CSF-2R [43].

One of the most promising targets are Janus Kinase (JAK) inhibitors which are pursuing to block the signaling pathways of cytokines. JAKs are kinases that are involved in the signaling of different cytokines. The JAK inhibitors would possibly block different cytokines at the same time. It will be interesting to see whether blocking JAKs in GCA artery will block the signaling of both vascular inflammation (IL6-mediated pathway) and vascular remodeling (IFNy-mediated pathway) at the same time. This very interesting concept was first demonstrated by the Weyand research group, by blocking concomitantly vascular inflammation and vascular remodeling, with tofacitinib (an inhibitor of Jak1 and 3) as shown in *ex vivo* studies by Zhang et al. 2017 [36]. SELECT-GCA is an ongoing Phase III clinical trial investigating Upadacitinib, another JAK inhibitor for active GCA, at new onset or relapse [43, 93].

4.3.3 Future therapeutical strategies and developments

In terms of therapeutic strategy, the question to ask is which targeted therapy has more GS-saving effects, and also which of them reduces vascular dysfunction and vascular remodeling, which is still the "unmet need" in GCA treatment. For these purposes, we could target by blocking different molecules for instance, endothelin 1, PDGF, mTor (rapamycin) [43]. TLR-induced activation of dendritic cells attracts and retain more dendritic cells and promote the activation of TH1 and TH17 cells, one of the putative therapeutic development would be TLR blockage [5]. vWF and its crosstalk with LRP4/integrin $\alpha_v\beta 3$ axis could also constitute a future target for new therapeutics (monoclonal antibody against VWF to prevent pathological hyperplasia of the GCA arterial wall [58], or as possible future research perspective and therapy objective one could investigate could be using a small molecule to inhibit Weibel-Palade bodies secretion from arterial ECs [82, 99] and therefore control ECs mediators' availability.

The impact of targeted GCA treatment on vascular inflammation and vascular remodeling, associated with vascular complications, needs to be further evaluated [22, 95] for more insight into the vascular inflammation and vascular repair unique features specific to GCA.

5. Discussion and conclusions

In this review study, we discussed several cellular and molecular pathogenetic mechanisms of vascular damage characteristic to GCA, that might occur during the progress of disease, especially during the active phase of the disease.

The paradigm in terms of GCA physiopathology is that inflammation starts in the adventitial layer with the activation of the vascular DCs which shifts the situation to the point where there are multiple types of immune cells recruited, proliferating, and differentiating in the vessel wall, causing together with inflamed vascular cells an erroneous repair of the arterial wall. It is unlikely that DCs are the one cells driving these processes, given the multitude of cell functions the arterial wall's ECs play in complicated processes of vascular inflammation, hemostasis/ thrombosis, and vascular repair, resulting in a distinct GCA-specific vasculopathy most commonly term used in the field is GCA-related vascular remodeling. There are three ECs populations in GCA artery: arterial luminal ECs, vasa vasorum ECs and capillary ECs formed *de novo* in the intima and media layers (which showed be avascular in a normal arteries) of the diseased artery. These three types of ECs are activated in a sequential manner, probably their activation is subordinated to the invading immune cells, but not to all. For instance, vasa vasorum ECs are activated after vascular DCs are activated but ECs activation most probably precedes the activation of T cells. The invading cells must get in the vessel wall through the vasa vasorum. Activated ECs provide the means for invasion by mobilizing, preformed contents of storage granules WPBs. These secreted ECs mediators are released in a timely manner to fulfill proinflammatory, chemoattractant and neoangiogenic roles, or increased endothelial permeability functions.

Biomarkers have the potential to detect the disease that is missed by TAB/imaging. Several large multi-centers clinical trials being done recently [43, 71, 95, 96] led to the discovery of new potential biomarkers to monitor disease activity and relapses, which is a new critical development in the field. Some of the recently published data imply that testing several blood acute phase reactants can optimize earlier diagnosis and the ability to predict flares and complications [73, 93].

In addition, our study underlines the importance of the candidate targets for novel therapeutics. In the more severe complications of this disease-as blindness or stroke-the underlying GCA-related vascular damage does not respond to GS, as previously reported by several independent studies. A multistep treatment for GCA should be envisioned which involves first line: steroids, especially when people with GCA are particular ill; and secondly, efficient medication to control vascular dysfunction (for instance to lower proinflammatory cytokine levels, to lower the levels of circulating active vWF in parallel). From the variety of GCA treatments that are being investigating a few have the potential to improve outcomes and reduce the need for steroids. The availability of new drug tocilizumab was received with a lot of enthusiasm it is the only FDA approved drug specific for GCA treatment. Tocilizumab is effective to control GCA symptoms, allows rapid GS tapering, and persistent remission with a low dose GS after 6 mo followup, however after tocilizumab discontinuation the relapse-free survival (%) decreases, at least in some patients. Tocilizumab poses certain challenges for clinicians regarding biomarkers follow-up of patients, since tocilizumab is repressing both CRP and ESR; therefore, making careful anamnesis, physical examination, and clinical judgement even more important part of the disease assessment. 20 adverse events were considered directly related to drug; danger with tocilizumab administration was reported in the instance of infection in patients receiving tocilizumab [43, 93], with pneumonia and no CRP and ESR rise, [43] signifying that more careful assessing of the disease activity and infections in the patients treated with tocilizumab is required [43]. Further studies are needed to determine the optimal duration of treatment and maintaining of dosing and to further reduce the risk of relapse [93]. An important note to make is that molecular pathogenic pathways promoting GCA disease are changing with the disease progression under treatment [93]. This situation is frequent in clinical practice and requires adequate follow-up and adapted therapeutic strategies [93].

Hopefully, future research will bring us closer to the goal of identifying new therapy for active and/or refractory GCA, which used in substitution or addition to steroids will provide tide control of the disease, addressing not only vascular inflammation but also vascular remodeling, skewed thrombotic propensity and luminal changes in GCA patients at the brink of having VL, or a stroke or other ischemic event at the initial onset of the arterial disease or in evolution.

Author details

Luiza Rusu
University of Illinois at Chicago, Chicago, Illinois, USA

*Address all correspondence to: luizarusu123@gmail.com

IntechOpen

References

[1] Hunder, G.G., et al., *The American College of Rheumatology 1990 criteria for the classification of giant cell arteritis.* Arthritis Rheum, 1990. **33**(8): p. 1122-8.

[2] Cid, M.C., et al., *Large vessel vasculitides.* Curr Opin Rheumatol, 1998. **10**(1): p. 18-28.

[3] Jennette, J.C., et al., *2012 revised International Chapel Hill Consensus Conference Nomenclature of Vasculitides.* Arthritis Rheum, 2013. **65**(1): p. 1-11.

[4] Weyand, C.M. and J.J. Goronzy, *Immune mechanisms in medium and large-vessel vasculitis.* Nat Rev Rheumatol, 2013. **9**(12): p. 731-40.

[5] Terrades-Garcia, N. and M.C. Cid, *Pathogenesis of giant-cell arteritis: how targeted therapies are influencing our understanding of the mechanisms involved.* Rheumatology (Oxford), 2018. **57**(suppl_2): p. ii51-ii62.

[6] Gonzalez-Gay, M.A., et al., *Giant cell arteritis: is the clinical spectrum of the disease changing?* BMC Geriatr, 2019. **19**(1): p. 200.

[7] Salvarani, C., et al., *Reappraisal of the epidemiology of giant cell arteritis in Olmsted County, Minnesota, over a fifty-year period.* Arthritis Rheum, 2004. **51**(2): p. 264-8.

[8] Mohammad, A.J., et al., *Rate of Comorbidities in Giant Cell Arteritis: A Population-based Study.* J Rheumatol, 2017. **44**(1): p. 84-90.

[9] Carmona, F.D., et al., *A Genome-wide Association Study Identifies Risk Alleles in Plasminogen and P4HA2 Associated with Giant Cell Arteritis.* Am J Hum Genet, 2017. **100**(1): p. 64-74.

[10] Weck, K.E., et al., *Murine gamma-herpesvirus 68 causes severe large-vessel arteritis in mice lacking interferon-gamma responsiveness: a new model for virus-induced vascular disease.* Nat Med, 1997. **3**(12): p. 1346-53.

[11] Deng, J., et al., *Toll-like receptors 4 and 5 induce distinct types of vasculitis.* Circ Res, 2009. **104**(4): p. 488-95.

[12] Ma-Krupa, W., et al., *Activation of arterial wall dendritic cells and breakdown of self-tolerance in giant cell arteritis.* J Exp Med, 2004. **199**(2): p. 173-83.

[13] Weyand, C.M., et al., *Tissue cytokine patterns in patients with polymyalgia rheumatica and giant cell arteritis.* Ann Intern Med, 1994. **121**(7): p. 484-91.

[14] Krupa, W.M., et al., *Trapping of misdirected dendritic cells in the granulomatous lesions of giant cell arteritis.* Am J Pathol, 2002. **161**(5): p. 1815-23.

[15] Baslund, B., et al., *Mortality in patients with giant cell arteritis.* Rheumatology (Oxford), 2015. **54**(1): p. 139-43.

[16] Klein, R.G., et al., *Skip lesions in temporal arteritis.* Mayo Clin Proc, 1976. **51**(8): p. 504-10.

[17] Kawasaki, A., et al., *Visualizing the skip lesions of giant cell arteritis with CT arteriography.* Eur Neurol, 2009. **61**(6): p. 374.

[18] Fraser, J.A., et al., *The treatment of giant cell arteritis.* Rev Neurol Dis, 2008. **5**(3): p. 140-52.

[19] Federici, A.B., et al., *Elevation of von Willebrand factor is independent of erythrocyte sedimentation rate and persists after glucocorticoid treatment in giant cell arteritis.* Arthritis Rheum, 1984. **27**(9): p. 1046-9.

[20] Persellin, S.T., et al., *Factor VIII-von Willebrand factor in giant cell arteritis and polymyalgia rheumatica.* Mayo Clin Proc, 1985. **60**(7): p. 457-62.

[21] Gonzalez-Gay, M.A., et al., *Treatment of giant cell arteritis.* Biochem Pharmacol, 2019. **165**: p. 230-239.

[22] Gonzalez-Gay, M.A. and T. Pina, *Giant cell arteritis and polymyalgia rheumatica: an update.* Curr Rheumatol Rep, 2015. **17**(2): p. 6.

[23] Cantini, F., et al., *Are polymyalgia rheumatica and giant cell arteritis the same disease?* Semin Arthritis Rheum, 2004. **33**(5): p. 294-301.

[24] de Boysson, H., et al., *Giant Cell Arteritis-related Stroke: A Retrospective Multicenter Case-control Study.* J Rheumatol, 2017. **44**(3): p. 297-303.

[25] Tomasson, G., et al., *Risk for cardiovascular disease early and late after a diagnosis of giant-cell arteritis: a cohort study.* Ann Intern Med, 2014. **160**(2): p. 73-80.

[26] Greigert, H., et al., *Myocardial infarction during giant cell arteritis: A cohort study.* Eur J Intern Med, 2021.

[27] Gonzalez-Gay, M.A., S. Castaneda, and J. Llorca, *Giant Cell Arteritis: Visual Loss Is Our Major Concern.* J Rheumatol, 2016. **43**(8): p. 1458-61.

[28] Gonzalez-Gay, M.A., et al., *Strokes at time of disease diagnosis in a series of 287 patients with biopsy-proven giant cell arteritis.* Medicine (Baltimore), 2009. **88**(4): p. 227-235.

[29] Proven, A., et al., *Glucocorticoid therapy in giant cell arteritis: duration and adverse outcomes.* Arthritis Rheum, 2003. **49**(5): p. 703-8.

[30] Calderon-Goercke, M., et al., *Tocilizumab in giant cell arteritis:*

differences between the GiACTA trial and a multicentre series of patients from the clinical practice. Clin Exp Rheumatol, 2020. **38 Suppl 124**(2): p. 112-119.

[31] Samson, M., et al., *Recent advances in our understanding of giant cell arteritis pathogenesis.* Autoimmun Rev, 2017. **16**(8): p. 833-844.

[32] Klein, M., et al., *[Giant cell arteritis with motor involvement of the upper trunk].* Nervenarzt, 2011. **82**(12): p. 1612-4.

[33] Gonzalez-Gay, M.A., et al., *Permanent visual loss and cerebrovascular accidents in giant cell arteritis: predictors and response to treatment.* Arthritis Rheum, 1998. **41**(8): p. 1497-504.

[34] Salvarani, C., F. Cantini, and G.G. Hunder, *Polymyalgia rheumatica and giant-cell arteritis.* Lancet, 2008. **372**(9634): p. 234-45.

[35] Ray, J.G., M.M. Mamdani, and W.H. Geerts, *Giant cell arteritis and cardiovascular disease in older adults.* Heart, 2005. **91**(3): p. 324-8.

[36] Zhang, H., et al., *Immunoinhibitory checkpoint deficiency in medium and large vessel vasculitis.* Proc Natl Acad Sci U S A, 2017. **114**(6): p. E970-E979.

[37] Wagner, A.D., et al., *Dendritic cells co-localize with activated CD4+ T cells in giant cell arteritis.* Clin Exp Rheumatol, 2003. **21**(2): p. 185-92.

[38] Deng, J., et al., *Th17 and Th1 T-cell responses in giant cell arteritis.* Circulation, 2010. **121**(7): p. 906-15.

[39] Conway, R., et al., *Ustekinumab for refractory giant cell arteritis: A prospective 52-week trial.* Semin Arthritis Rheum, 2018. **48**(3): p. 523-528.

[40] Conway, R. and E.S. Molloy, *Ustekinumab in Giant Cell Arteritis.*

Comment on the Article by Matza et al. Arthritis Care Res (Hoboken), 2020.

[41] Miyabe, C., et al., *An expanded population of pathogenic regulatory T cells in giant cell arteritis is abrogated by IL-6 blockade therapy.* Ann Rheum Dis, 2017. **76**(5): p. 898-905.

[42] Hernandez-Rodriguez, J., et al., *Elevated production of interleukin-6 is associated with a lower incidence of disease-related ischemic events in patients with giant-cell arteritis: angiogenic activity of interleukin-6 as a potential protective mechanism.* Circulation, 2003. **107**(19): p. 2428-34.

[43] Samson, M., et al., *Biological treatments in giant cell arteritis & Takayasu arteritis.* Eur J Intern Med, 2018. **50**: p. 12-19.

[44] Hilhorst, M., et al., *T cell-macrophage interactions and granuloma formation in vasculitis.* Front Immunol, 2014. **5**: p. 432.

[45] Cid, M.C., et al., *Association between increased CCL2 (MCP-1) expression in lesions and persistence of disease activity in giant-cell arteritis.* Rheumatology (Oxford), 2006. **45**(11): p. 1356-63.

[46] Corbera-Bellalta, M., et al., *Blocking interferon gamma reduces expression of chemokines CXCL9, CXCL10 and CXCL11 and decreases macrophage infiltration in ex vivo cultured arteries from patients with giant cell arteritis.* Ann Rheum Dis, 2016. **75**(6): p. 1177-86.

[47] Samson, M., et al., *Involvement and prognosis value of CD8(+) T cells in giant cell arteritis.* J Autoimmun, 2016. **72**: p. 73-83.

[48] Wagner, A.D., J.J. Goronzy, and C.M. Weyand, *Functional profile of tissue-infiltrating and circulating CD68+ cells in giant cell arteritis. Evidence for two components of the disease.* J Clin Invest, 1994. **94**(3): p. 1134-40.

[49] Weyand, C.M., et al., *Correlation of the topographical arrangement and the functional pattern of tissue-infiltrating macrophages in giant cell arteritis.* J Clin Invest, 1996. **98**(7): p. 1642-9.

[50] Kaiser, M., et al., *Platelet-derived growth factor, intimal hyperplasia, and ischemic complications in giant cell arteritis.* Arthritis Rheum, 1998. **41**(4): p. 623-33.

[51] Lozano, E., et al., *Imatinib mesylate inhibits in vitro and ex vivo biological responses related to vascular occlusion in giant cell arteritis.* Ann Rheum Dis, 2008. **67**(11): p. 1581-8.

[52] Baldini, M., et al., *Selective up-regulation of the soluble pattern-recognition receptor pentraxin 3 and of vascular endothelial growth factor in giant cell arteritis: relevance for recent optic nerve ischemia.* Arthritis Rheum, 2012. **64**(3): p. 854-65.

[53] Hafner, F., et al., *Endothelial function and carotid intima-media thickness in giant-cell arteritis.* Eur J Clin Invest, 2014. **44**(3): p. 249-56.

[54] Watanabe, R., et al., *MMP (Matrix Metalloprotease)-9-Producing Monocytes Enable T Cells to Invade the Vessel Wall and Cause Vasculitis.* Circ Res, 2018. **123**(6): p. 700-715.

[55] Cid, M.C., et al., *Cell adhesion molecules in the development of inflammatory infiltrates in giant cell arteritis: inflammation-induced angiogenesis as the preferential site of leukocyte-endothelial cell interactions.* Arthritis Rheum, 2000. **43**(1): p. 184-94.

[56] Rittner, H.L., et al., *Tissue-destructive macrophages in giant cell arteritis.* Circ Res, 1999. **84**(9): p. 1050-8.

[57] Segarra, M., et al., *Gelatinase expression and proteolytic activity in*

giant-cell arteritis. Ann Rheum Dis, 2007. **66**(11): p. 1429-35.

[58] Lagrange, J., et al., *The VWF/LRP4/ alphaVbeta3-axis represents a novel pathway regulating proliferation of human vascular smooth muscle cells.* Cardiovasc Res, 2021.

[59] Murray, P.I., et al., *Von Willebrand factor, endothelial damage and ocular disease.* Ocul Immunol Inflamm, 1993. **1**(4): p. 315-22.

[60] Qin, F., et al., *Overexpression of von Willebrand factor is an independent risk factor for pathogenesis of intimal hyperplasia: preliminary studies.* J Vasc Surg, 2003. **37**(2): p. 433-9.

[61] Gaffo, A.L., *Thrombosis in vasculitis.* Best Pract Res Clin Rheumatol, 2013. **27**(1): p. 57-67.

[62] Kaiser, M., et al., *Formation of new vasa vasorum in vasculitis. Production of angiogenic cytokines by multinucleated giant cells.* Am J Pathol, 1999. **155**(3): p. 765-74.

[63] Lozano, E., et al., *Increased expression of the endothelin system in arterial lesions from patients with giant-cell arteritis: association between elevated plasma endothelin levels and the development of ischaemic events.* Ann Rheum Dis, 2010. **69**(2): p. 434-42.

[64] Planas-Rigol, E., et al., *Endothelin-1 promotes vascular smooth muscle cell migration across the artery wall: a mechanism contributing to vascular remodelling and intimal hyperplasia in giant-cell arteritis.* Ann Rheum Dis, 2017. **76**(9): p. 1624-1634.

[65] Zeiffer, U., et al., *Neointimal smooth muscle cells display a proinflammatory phenotype resulting in increased leukocyte recruitment mediated by P-selectin and chemokines.* Circ Res, 2004. **94**(6): p. 776-84.

[66] Avina-Zubieta, J.A., et al., *The risk of deep venous thrombosis and pulmonary embolism in giant cell arteritis: a general population-based study.* Ann Rheum Dis, 2016. **75**(1): p. 148-54.

[67] Gonzalez-Gay, M.A., et al., *Biopsy-proven giant cell arteritis patients with coronary artery disease have increased risk of aortic aneurysmal disease and arterial thrombosis.* Clin Exp Rheumatol, 2013. **31**(1 Suppl 75): p. S94.

[68] Tsoukas, A., et al., *Clinically Apparent Arterial Thrombosis in Persons with Systemic Vasculitis.* Int J Rheumatol, 2017. **2017**: p. 3572768.

[69] Weyand, C.M., et al., *Therapeutic effects of acetylsalicylic acid in giant cell arteritis.* Arthritis Rheum, 2002. **46**(2): p. 457-66.

[70] Stone, J.H., *Antiplatelet versus anticoagulant therapy in patients with giant cell arteritis: which is best?* Nat Clin Pract Rheumatol, 2007. **3**(3): p. 136-7.

[71] Samson, M. and B. Bonnotte, *Ustekinumab for the treatment of giant cell arteritis: Comment on the paper of Martza et al.* Arthritis Care Res (Hoboken), 2020.

[72] Wojcik, B.M., et al., *Interleukin-6: a potential target for post-thrombotic syndrome.* Ann Vasc Surg, 2011. **25**(2): p. 229-39.

[73] Hocevar, A., et al., *Do Early Diagnosis and Glucocorticoid Treatment Decrease the Risk of Permanent Visual Loss and Early Relapses in Giant Cell Arteritis: A Prospective Longitudinal Study.* Medicine (Baltimore), 2016. **95**(14): p. e3210.

[74] Luther, R., et al., *Increased number of cases of giant cell arteritis and higher rates of ophthalmic involvement during the era of COVID-19.* Rheumatol Adv Pract, 2020. **4**(2): p. rkaa067.

[75] Salvarani, C., et al., *Endothelial nitric oxide synthase gene polymorphisms in giant cell arteritis*. Arthritis Rheum, 2003. **48**(11): p. 3219-23.

[76] Subramaniam, M., et al., *Defects in hemostasis in P-selectin-deficient mice*. Blood, 1996. **87**(4): p. 1238-42.

[77] Garcia, J.G., et al., *Thrombin-induced increase in albumin permeability across the endothelium*. J Cell Physiol, 1986. **128**(1): p. 96-104.

[78] Chen, D. and A. Dorling, *Critical roles for thrombin in acute and chronic inflammation*. J Thromb Haemost, 2009. **7 Suppl 1**: p. 122-6.

[79] Coughlin, S.R., *Protease-activated receptors in hemostasis, thrombosis and vascular biology*. J Thromb Haemost, 2005. **3**(8): p. 1800-14.

[80] Vu, T.K., et al., *Molecular cloning of a functional thrombin receptor reveals a novel proteolytic mechanism of receptor activation*. Cell, 1991. **64**(6): p. 1057-68.

[81] Kaufman, D.P., T. Sanvictores, and M. Costanza, *Weibel Palade Bodies*, in *StatPearls*. 2021: Treasure Island (FL).

[82] Rusu, L., et al., *G protein-dependent basal and evoked endothelial cell vWF secretion*. Blood, 2014. **123**(3): p. 442-50.

[83] Springer, J. and A. Villa-Forte, *Thrombosis in vasculitis*. Curr Opin Rheumatol, 2013. **25**(1): p. 19-25.

[84] Schillemans, M., et al., *Exocytosis of Weibel-Palade bodies: how to unpack a vascular emergency kit*. J Thromb Haemost, 2019. **17**(1): p. 6-18.

[85] Gragnano, F., et al., *The Role of von Willebrand Factor in Vascular Inflammation: From Pathogenesis to Targeted Therapy*. Mediators Inflamm, 2017. **2017**: p. 5620314.

[86] Cossutta, M., et al., *Weibel-Palade Bodies Orchestrate Pericytes During Angiogenesis*. Arterioscler Thromb Vasc Biol, 2019. **39**(9): p. 1843-1858.

[87] Woodburn, K.R., et al., *Fibrinogen and markers of fibrinolysis and endothelial damage following resolution of critical limb ischaemia*. Eur J Vasc Endovasc Surg, 1995. **10**(3): p. 272-8.

[88] Fuster, V. and E.J. Bowie, *The von Willebrand pig as a model for atherosclerosis research*. Thromb Haemost, 1978. **39**(2): p. 322-7.

[89] Mohan, S.V., et al., *Giant cell arteritis: immune and vascular aging as disease risk factors*. Arthritis Res Ther, 2011. **13**(4): p. 231.

[90] Gonzalez-Gay, M.A., et al., *Giant cell arteritis: more than a cranial disease*. Clin Exp Rheumatol, 2020. **38 Suppl 124**(2): p. 15-17.

[91] Soriano, A., et al., *Visual loss and other cranial ischaemic complications in giant cell arteritis*. Nat Rev Rheumatol, 2017. **13**(8): p. 476-484.

[92] Maleszewski, J.J., et al., *Clinical and pathological evolution of giant cell arteritis: a prospective study of follow-up temporal artery biopsies in 40 treated patients*. Mod Pathol, 2017. **30**(6): p. 788-796.

[93] Serling-Boyd, N. and J.H. Stone, *Recent advances in the diagnosis and management of giant cell arteritis*. Curr Opin Rheumatol, 2020. **32**(3): p. 201-207.

[94] Stone, J.H., et al., *Trial of Tocilizumab in Giant-Cell Arteritis*. N Engl J Med, 2017. **377**(4): p. 317-328.

[95] Stone, J.H., et al., *Glucocorticoid Dosages and Acute-Phase Reactant Levels at Giant Cell Arteritis Flare in a Randomized Trial of Tocilizumab*. Arthritis Rheumatol, 2019. **71**(8): p. 1329-1338.

[96] Langford, C.A., et al., *A Randomized, Double-Blind Trial of Abatacept (CTLA-4Ig) for the Treatment of Takayasu Arteritis.* Arthritis Rheumatol, 2017. **69**(4): p. 846-853.

[97] Conway, R., et al., *Ustekinumab for the treatment of refractory giant cell arteritis.* Ann Rheum Dis, 2016. **75**(8): p. 1578-9.

[98] Matza, M.A., et al., *Ustekinumab for the Treatment of Giant Cell Arteritis.* Arthritis Care Res (Hoboken), 2020.

[99] Rusu, L., Minshall R. D., *Composition and Method for Treating Thrombosis.* US Patent, 2018.

Chapter 3

Extra-Cranial Involvement in Giant Cell Arteritis

João Fernandes Serôdio, Miguel Trindade, Catarina Favas and José Delgado Alves

Abstract

Recent advances in imaging studies and treatment approaches have greatly improved our knowledge about Giant Cell Arteritis (GCA). Previously thought of as a predominantly cranial disease, we now know that GCA is a systemic disease that may involve other medium and large vessel territories. Several imaging studies have shown that between 30 and 70% of patients with GCA present with large-vessel vasculitis. Moreover, a significant proportion of patients present large-vessel disease in the absence of cranial involvement. Extra-cranial disease also poses management challenges as these patients may have a more refractory-relapsing disease course and need additional therapies. Aortic dilation and aneurysms are well-described late complications of GCA involving the large artery territories. In this chapter, we discuss the clinical picture of extra-cranial involvement in GCA, focusing on improved diagnostic protocols and suitable treatment strategies.

Keywords: giant cell arteritis, large-vessel vasculitis, polymyalgia rheumatica, vasculitis, diagnostic imaging

1. Introduction

Giant cell arteritis (GCA) is a systemic vasculitis that predominantly involves large and medium-size arteries [1]. It occurs almost exclusively in subjects aged 50 years or older, and is the most common form of systemic vasculitis among the elderly [2]. GCA is more common among caucasian female patients, with a female–male ratio of about 2–3:1. The GCA annual incidence varies with geographical location and ranges from 1.6 to 32.8 cases/100000 persons ≥50 years of age [3].

GCA is commonly defined as Large-Vessel (LV) GCA if the aorta and its branches are involved. The systemic nature of the disease was noted as early as the first cases described by Horton and colleagues in 1932 [4]. Later on, Gilmour suggested that the disease should be called "giant-cell chronic arteritis" as the temporal arteritis appeared to be only part of a more widespread vascular disease [5]. Despite this early reports, physicians have mainly focused on typical cranial symptoms and visual disturbances and have relied mostly on temporal biopsy for diagnosis. This focus is well reflected in the 1990 ACR classification criteria that emphasised the importance of headache as a cardinal symptom and temporal biopsy as its primary diagnostic tool [6]. Unfortunately, the concept of GCA as a limited cranial disease is inaccurate and obscures essential clinical features. Furthermore, the misuse of classification criteria for diagnostic purposes, may lead to underdiagnose LV-GCA [7].

In recent years there has been an increased awareness of the systemic large-artery nature of GCA. Necropsy studies have shown histologic evidence of systemic large-artery vasculitis in approximately 80% of patients [8, 9]. Recent advances in diagnostic imaging techniques have confirmed these figures, suggesting that imaging will have an increasing impact in the diagnosis and management of GCA [10–14]. Furthermore, patients with GCA are at increased risk of developing aortic dilation and aneurysms among other complications [15–17].

Altogether, these issues highlight the importance of the extra-cranial involvement of GCA which has been under-recognised and poorly managed.

2. Pathophysiology

GCA is an idiopathic inflammatory granulomatous vasculitis. The aetiology is unknown, and most probably, genetic, environmental, vascular, and age-related factors concur to the development of the disease [2, 18]. In GCA, a lymphocyte and plasma cell infiltrate originates at the *vasa vasorum* in the adventitia of large vessels, which then penetrates the vessel wall leading to an intimal and media hyperplasia and vessel wall thickening [19]. Multinucleated giant cells form a complex near the intima-media complex, but they are not a requisite for diagnosis. Inflammation can be segmental, circumferential, or transmural [9, 20]. The predominance of GCA by some vessel territories and the mechanisms behind the different phenotypes like LV-GCA are still unsolved questions. In fact, most studies have been performed in temporal artery biopsies, as large arteries are not as readily accessible for histologic examination. Animal models also present limitations regarding the expression of the disease in different vascular territories. The interaction of immunopathogenic mechanisms with the different functional and anatomic characteristics of the vessel walls in different parts of the body may explain the distinct aspects of LV-GCA pathophysiology.

2.1 Immunologic mechanisms in large vessel giant cell arteritis

The critical event in initiating and sustaining the inflammatory response is thought to be the abnormal maturation and loss of tolerance of vascular Ddendritic cells (DCs), which is triggered by toll-like receptors (TLRs) [21, 22]. Differentiated DCs drive T cell and macrophage recruitment [21]. Upon the maturation of DCs, CD4+ T cells are also stimulated by local cytokines, such as IL12, to polarise into T-helper 1 (Th1) and IL6 and IL23 to polarise into Th17 cells [23].

TH17 cells are responsible for implementing a strong acute IL17 mediated inflammatory response, which leads to the overproduction of a cluster of cytokines, namely IL1β, IL6, IL23 and TNF-α [23]. Type II cytokine receptors (mainly IL6 and IL1β) signal through JAK1 homo-dimers [24] promoting further cellular activation and inflammatory response. The IL17 pathway is therefore responsible for most of the inflammatory response in the acute phase and explains the systemic nature of the disease [25, 26].

Th1 cells differentiation induces an immune response where IFN-γ is the central cytokine [27]. IFN-γ receptor signals through JAK1–JAK2 heterodimers [28]. The INF-γ signature further enhances the inflammatory response (through IL1β, IL6, and TNF-α), leading to macrophage differentiation and activation. Upon the stimulation by the granulocyte-macrophage colony-stimulating factor (GM-CSF) produced by T cells, macrophages act in sustaining inflammation and are key players in the interaction with the stromal and extracellular matrix [29, 30]. This interaction is mediated by matrix metalloproteinases (MMP) and several growth factors.

MMP are proteases with elastolytic activity, released and activated by inflammatory cells. Smooth muscle loss and proteolytic imbalance may contribute to elastic
fibre rupture, weakening of the artery wall, and cell migration [29, 31]. The IFN-γ
signature is responsible for the histiocytic reaction, myofibroblast differentiation,
intimal hyperplasia, neoangiogenesis, vascular remodelling, damage, and fibrosis
[32]. These aspects explain the vascular manifestations and the LV complications
of GCA. Current treatments efficiently inhibit the Th17-mediated response, but
not the Th1 mediated expression of IFN-γ [27, 33]. Thus, the current management
of vascular manifestations like artery stenosis and aneurysms is suboptimal, as
vascular remodelling processes may subsist even in the absence of raised inflammatory markers [34].

Patients with polymyalgia rheumatica (PMR) present activated DCs in focal
vessel infiltrates with the expression of inflammatory cytokine production (IL1β
and IL6), but IFN-y is absent [35]. Therefore, it is thought that it is the IFN-γ pathway, and not IL17 activation that marks the progression to overt vascular inflammation and remodelling.

It is not yet clear why some patients have only PMR while others progress to
periadventitial or transmural vasculitis. Different TLR expression on DCs may
partly explain such patterns as TLR4 activation induces transmural panarteritis,
while TLR5 ligands promote adventitial perivasculitis [36]. Moreover, DCs exhibit
distinct combinations of TLRs in different vascular beds [37]. Thus, the phenotype
of the vasculitis may depend upon the profile of the TLR driven T cell activation,
which is specific of each vascular territory.

The interaction between T cells and B cells might also be implicated in the
expression of LV-GCA. Recent findings in aorta tissue samples from 9 LV-GCA
patients who underwent aortic aneurysm surgery, showed massive infiltration of
B-cells, which outnumbered T-cells. B-cells were mainly found in the adventitia and
were organised into tertiary lymphoid organs [38]. This is an uncommon observation in temporal artery biopsies.

The interaction of immune mechanisms and the vascular matrix is also demonstrated by the MMP expression in singular vascular fields. MMP2 tissue expression
was observed in active temporal artery lesions and in aortic aneurysm samples
obtained in 2 GCA patients. However, MMP9 was present only in temporal artery
lesions and faintly detectable in normal temporal arteries and GCA-related aneurysms [17]. While MMP9 is mainly produced by inflammatory cells, MMP2 may
also be expressed in smooth muscle cells and be involved in reparative mechanisms.
Therefore, the expression of MMPs on different vascular beds may also impact on
the clinical features of GCA.

2.2 Atherosclerosis, ageing and large vessel vasculitis

Atherosclerosis is highly prevalent among GCA patients as it is most present at
an advanced age. The coexistence of these two diseases and the underlying immune
mechanisms of both may tailor the phenotype of the vasculitis. It is known that
patients with cardiovascular risk factors have a higher risk of developing severe
ischaemic manifestations of GCA [39]. In fact, patients with ischemic complications
have lower expression of IL6 suggesting that IL6 may play a protective angiogenic
role to compensate for ischemia [40]. Furthermore, at the supra-aortic level,
atherosclerosis most commonly affects the carotids, while LV-GCA predominantly
affects the axillary arteries. Regardless of the immune profile, age and genetic
factors also influence the development of atherosclerosis. In caucasians, atherosclerosis occurs later and less extensively in intracranial arteries compared to extra-
cranial arteries. Interestingly, Asian and African populations are more affected by

intracranial atherosclerosis and also show a low prevalence of cranial GCA [3, 41]. Thus, atherosclerosis may alter vessel vulnerability or expression of GCA.

Age is an important factor that affects vascular and immune processes with a possible impact on disease vulnerability and manifestations [42]. Ageing induces significant changes in the expression of vascular MMP2 and MMP9 and reduces arterial smooth muscle proliferative capacity [43–45]. One of the main distinctions between LV-GCA and Takayasu arteritis (TAK) has been attributed to an age cut-off. Interestingly, TAK shows similar immunologic mechanisms with dysregulated activation of Th1 and Th17 pathways [46] and therefore age-related factors may be the key to explain the distinct manifestations between LV-GCA and TAK [20, 42].

3. Clinical features of large vessel giant cell arteritis

3.1 Clinical manifestations

LV-GCA usually presents with prominent constitutional symptoms and a marked increase in inflammatory markers. Systemic constitutional symptoms include fever, malaise, weight loss and night sweats. Symptoms are usually non-specific and, in up to 20% of the patients, systemic constitutional symptoms are the only clinical features of the disease with some cases being diagnosed following an investigation for fever of unknown origin [10, 18]. Aortitis is a common feature in LV-GCA. Aortitis is often pauci-symptomatic, but some patients may refer chest or back pain [18]. LV-GCA also affects the main arteries of the limbs, presenting most commonly as limb claudication. Limb claudication reflects intimal and muscular hyperplasia secondary to vascular inflammation, which leads to vessel wall thickening with lumen occlusion. Limb claudication involves the arms more frequently than the legs and may be present in up to 50% of LV-GCA patients. It can be intermittent and asymmetric despite vascular involvement being bilateral in around 80% of the patients [7, 10, 47].

The preferred vascular territories involved are the supra-aortic branches, particularly the axillary and subclavian arteries, which are involved in almost all patients with LV-GCA. Carotid and vertebral artery involvement are less frequent. Aortitis is present in around 50–65% of the patients with documented LV-GCA. Most commonly, it involves the aortic arch and the thoracic descending aorta. When the abdominal aorta is affected, there is usually involvement of the thoracic segment as well. Femoral arteries and inferior limb arteries are involved in only around 10–15% of the patients. Sometimes differential diagnosis with atherosclerosis, very commonly found in these arteries, may be difficult. Visceral arteries are rarely affected [7, 10, 12, 47–49].

3.2 Clinical overlap between large vessel vasculitis, cranial giant cell arteritis and polymyalgia rheumatica

There is a considerable clinical and epidemiologic overlap between GCA and PMR. PMR is a clinical syndrome characterised by bilateral shoulder pain, morning stiffness, shoulder or pelvic girdle weakness, and peripheral arthralgia/arthritis [2]. Approximately 20% of PMR patients have GCA, whereas PMR is present in up to 60% of GCA patients [2, 50, 51]. PMR is also the main form of relapse in up to 50% of GCA patients, while cranial symptoms are relatively uncommon at relapse [52]. Interestingly, Positron Emission Tomography ([18]FDG-PET) LV fluorodeoxyglucose increased uptake was noted in 30% of patients with isolated polymyalgia rheumatica at diagnosis [53]. Therefore, PMR patients with incomplete response to corticosteroid treatment or a relapsing disease should be re-evaluated for LV involvement.

Patients with LV-GCA are more frequently women and present at a younger age, whereas patients with cranial GCA are usually men and older [7, 10, 54]. When compared with cranial GCA, patients with LV-GCA present less frequently with headache (35% in LV-GCA vs. 60% in cranial GCA), jaw claudication (22% in LV-GCA vs. 50% in cranial GCA) and also with fewer cranial ischemic symptoms (permanent visual loss in 4% in LV-GCA vs. 20% in cranial GCA) [10, 55–57]. Although there may be specificities concerning the presentation of cranial GCA and LV-GCA, they are not distinct entities (**Table 1**). More likely, we are facing a different spectrum of the same disease (**Figure 1**). Depending on the different imaging techniques used, 32–83% of the patients with confirmed cranial GCA also have LV vasculitis [10–12, 14] and 10–30% of the patients with GCA have only LV vasculitis, with no clinical, histologic or Doppler evidence of temporal artery vasculitis [10, 48, 58, 59].

Symptoms and signs	Cranial GCA	LV-GCA	PMR
Headache	+ +	+	—
Jaw claudication	+ +	—	—
Visual disturbances	+ +	—	—
Limb claudication	+	+ +	—
Fever, night sweats, weight loss	+	+ +	+
Polymyalgic symptoms	+	+ +	+ +
Peripheral arthralgia/arthritis	+	+	+ +
Elevation of inflammatory markers	+ +	+ +	+ +

GCA, Giant Cell Arteritis; LV, Large Vessel; PMR, Polymyalgia Rheumatica; –, uncommon symptom or sign;
+, common symptom or sign; ++, very common symptom or sign.

Table 1.
Clinical symptoms and signs in different subtypes of GCA and in PMR.

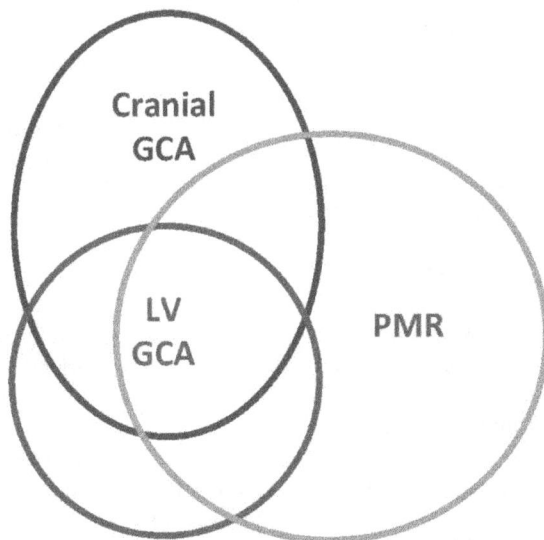

Figure 1.
The clinical spectrum of cranial GCA, LV-GCA and PMR.

Due to the more unspecific nature of the clinical presentation of LV-GCA, the diagnosis is often delayed or even missed. In general, patients with isolated LV-GCA have a delay in the diagnosis greater than one year compared with patients with cranial GCA [7]. It is still unknown whether this delay in diagnosis and treatment may impact the clinical course of the disease. However, LV-GCA patients relapse more frequently and earlier than those with cranial GCA and have higher corticosteroid cumulative doses and more frequently require additional immunosuppressive treatments [7, 54]. These facts suggest that patients with LV-GCA should be considered for a different management and treatment strategy, with a more tailored, eventually more aggressive approach.

4. Differential diagnosis

The systemic LV involvement in GCA may resemble the presentation of Takayasu arteritis (TAK). Patients with Takayasu's disease may present with raised inflammatory markers, vascular bruits, asymmetric blood pressure measurements and limb claudication, much like patients with LV-GCA. The recent widening of the concept of vascular involvement in GCA shows that there can be an overlap between these two conditions. However, some have proposed clear distinctions. Most importantly, the epidemiology is quite different. GCA is recurrent among northern European patients, whereas TAK is more prevalent among the Asian population [60]. Another difference is the age of disease onset. GCA is almost exclusively present in patients 50 years or older, whereas TAK is common under 40 [2, 61]. However, some argue age restriction to be arbitrary and without etiologic or pathophysiologic basis [20]. In a study of 96 Japanese patients with TAK, 22% were outside the proposed age cut-off [62]. Likewise, in the study that defined the 1990 ACR Classification Criteria for GCA, 23% of the patients had less than 50 years old at diagnosis [6]. Moreover, these definitions are elusive for patients with LV vasculitis aged between 40 and 50 years. So, distinguishing GCA and TAK based only on age and epidemiology may be difficult suggesting that we might, in fact, be looking at two forms of the same disease [63].

The histopathologic findings in both GCA and TAK show a lymphohistiocytic infiltrate in the vascular wall that may be indistinguishable [20]. However, this observation may be biased due to the small number of patients undergoing vascular biopsy in TAK. Pathophysiologic mechanisms also show common features between both diseases [42, 46]. Clinically, TAK presents with a more widespread vascular involvement. The carotid and mesenteric arteries are more frequently affected in patients with TAK than GCA, while subclavian and axillary artery involvement is more prevalent in LV-GCA [63, 64]. The aortic involvement is also distinct since stenotic/occlusive lesions are predominant in TAK, whereas aneurysmal disease is more common in GCA [64]. It is unclear, however, if the differences in imaging findings represent cumulative damage due to delay in TAK diagnosis or whether other age-related immunologic and vascular factors may explain these differences. Lastly, inflammatory markers seem to be higher in patients with GCA than in TAK. Around 44% of the patients with TAK may have active vascular inflammation despite normal inflammatory marker values [65].

Several cases of small and medium vessel vasculitis have been described with temporal artery involvement, particularly granulomatosis with polyangiitis and eosinophilic granulomatosis with polyangiitis [66]. However, the presentation of ANCA-associated vasculitis with aortitis is extremely rare [67] and even more so in other forms of primary vasculitis.

Infectious diseases	Immune-mediated diseases
Syphilis aortitis	**Systemic vasculitis**
Salmonella spp	Takayasu Arteritis
Staphylococcus spp	ANCA-associated vasculitis
Micobacterium tuberculosis	Panarteritis nodosa
Sub-acute endocarditis	**Autoimmune diseases**
Haematological and oncological disorders	Systemic lupus erythematosus
Erdheim-Chester histiocytosis	Rheumatoid arthritis
Amyloidosis	**Inflammatory diseases**
Paraneoplastic retroperitoneal fibrosis	HLA-B27 associated spondyloarthropathies
Vascular disease	Behçet disease
Atherosclerosis	Cogan disease
	Relapsing polychondritis
	Other
	Idiopathic aortitis
	IgG4-related disease
	Sarcoidosis

Table 2.
Differential diagnosis of large-vessel giant cell arteritis.

Other systemic diseases present with aortitis and may also be mistaken with LV-GCA (**Table 2**). Some infections like syphilis or sub-acute endocarditis may evolve with aortitis [68, 69]. In these cases, serologic and microbiologic studies often guide the diagnosis. Other immune-mediated diseases also have aortitis as a prominent clinical feature such as Behçets disease, IgG4-related disease, and Erdheim-Chester disease. These entities often have other distinctive organ involvement and typical histologic findings pointing to a different diagnosis [69–71]. Also, in IgG4-related and Erdheim-Chester diseases, aortic involvement occurs as peri-aortitis and retroperitoneal fibrosis which is different from vascular inflammation. Aortitis may also be a late complication of ankylosing spondylitis. It often involves de aortic root or the iliac periaortic peritoneum. It presents late in the disease, and articular symptoms often precede it by years. With recent advances in treatment, it is expected that it will become a less common manifestation of the disease [72].

5. Imaging features of large-vessel giant cell arteritis

Several imaging techniques have contributed to significant improvements in the assessment and management of LV-GCA, yet no single method is considered preferable (**Table 3**).

5.1 Ultrasonography

Ultrasonography has become widely used in GCA as it can be comparable to biopsy in the diagnosis of temporal arteritis [48, 73]. The presence of a regular hypoechoic non-compressible area around the lumen (the "halo sign") that reflects an oedematous inflammatory intima-media thickening is considered diagnostic of medium and large vessel vasculitis [74]. It is distinguished from atherosclerotic plaques since atherosclerosis presents as irregular iso- or hyper-echoic extrusions. Ultrasonography identifies aspects compatible with LV-GCA in 29–48% of patients when axillary-subclavian arteries are systematically analysed, and this standard evaluation is particularly important as 13–33% of patients have LV-GCA in the absence of temporal involvement [10, 11, 48, 58, 59]. The identification in the axillary arteries of a smooth hypoechoic increase in the intima-media thickness (IMT)

Imaging technique	Findings of LV vasculitis	GCA with LV vasculitis	Diagnostic accuracy under treatment
Ultrasonography	• Hypoechoic wall thickening (halo)	29–48% [10, 48, 58, 59]	2 weeks
CT and CTA	• Circumferential wall thickening • Wall contrast enhancement.	45–68% [12, 77, 78]	3 days
MRI	• Circumferential wall thickening • T2 sequence enhanced wall oedema	~54% [82]	—
^{18}FDG-PET	• Increase vascular ^{18}FDG uptake	58–83% [14, 49, 83]	10 days

CT, Computed tomography; CTA, CT angiography; MRI, magnetic resonance; ^{18}FDG-PET, ^{8}F-deoxyglucose positron emission tomography; –, unavailable data.

Table 3.
Imaging methods in the diagnosis of large vessel inflammation in giant cell arteritis.

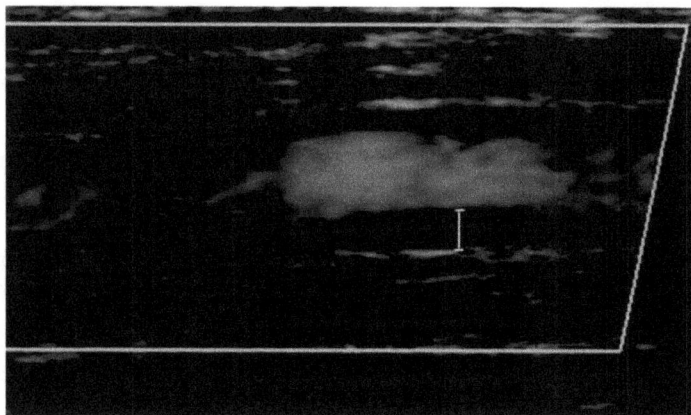

Figure 2.
Doppler ultrasonography of a right axillary artery in a patient with Large Vessel Giant Cell Arteritis. White line shows a smoothly increased hypo-echoic intima-media thickness of around 1.5 mm.

(with a local cut-off for IMT ≥1 mm) correctly identified LV-GCA (**Figure 2**) with a sensitivity and a specificity of close to 100% [75].

Ultrasonography has the advantage of being inexpensive, not using ionising radiation and can be readily accessible to use, as demonstrated in the implementation of fast track clinics [55, 57], though it requires experienced sonographers. Ultrasonography may also be useful in disease monitoring, as most patients show the disappearance of wall thickening over the course of steroid treatment [76]. This is why ultrasonographic signs are accurate for diagnosis purposes only within the first two weeks of corticosteroid treatment, losing sensitivity thereafter [74, 76], whilst thoracic aorta examination is not easily accessible by ultrasound.

5.2 Computed tomography

Computed tomography (CT) and CT angiography (CTA) are useful for LV imaging: they have a short scanning time yet allowing for a comprehensive vascular assessment, including the thoracic and abdominal aorta. Prospective studies of newly diagnosed

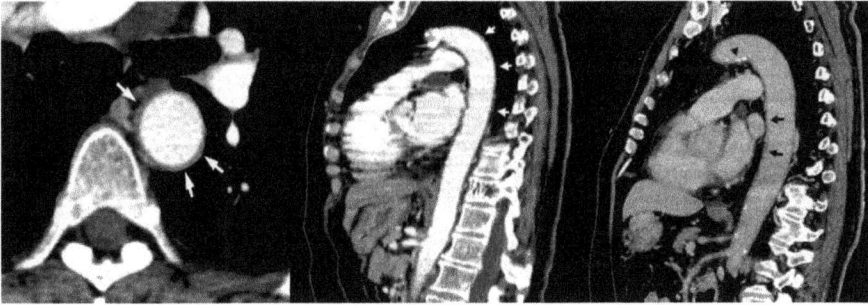

Figure 3.
Computed tomography (CT) and CT angiography (CTA) revealing Large Vessel Vasculitis in Giant Cell Arteritis (GCA). Left image shows a CTA image with circumferential wall thickening >2 mm of the thoracic aorta. Central CTA image shows the extent of thoracic aorta wall thickening in the same patient, predominantly involving posterior wall. Right image reveals thoracic wall thickening in CT of another GCA patient. Arrow depicts vasculitic wall thickening, arrowhead depicts atherosclerotic calcified plaque.

GCA patients assessed by CTA have revealed LV involvement in 45–68% of subjects [12, 77, 78]. Typical findings of LV include circumferential wall thickening and vessel wall contrast enhancement. However, CTA findings may be attenuated by an as short as three-day course of corticosteroid treatment [12]. Nevertheless, up to 43% of patients still present significant arterial wall thickening one year after treatment [79]. The simultaneous assessment of aortic dilation and the adequate distinction between vasculitis and atherosclerosis, which appears as focal calcifications, are other advantages of CTA. Ionising radiation is of concern when repetitive evaluations are performed, but novel low-dose CTA techniques may reduce radiation exposure (**Figure 3**) [80].

5.3 Magnetic resonance

Magnetic Resonance (MRI) conveys a wide vascular assessment with vasculitis appearing as a mural thickening or wall oedema, enhanced in T2 sequences. High-resolution MRI has been extensively used to assess temporal arteritis, but there is little experience with MRI in LV-GCA [13, 81, 82]. In contrast, and as MRI does not require iodinated contrast or ionising radiation, it has been exhaustively used for periodic assessment in younger patients with TAK [80].

5.4 Positron emission tomography

[18]FDG-PET has become widely used in LV-GCA as it allows broad vascular assessment of inflamed vascular territories that have an increased glucose metabolism. Accordingly, 58–83% of patients with GCA show LV involvement in [18]FDG-PET studies [14, 49, 83]. [18]FDG-PET also has the advantage of suggesting possible differential diagnoses such as infectious or neoplastic disease. However, it is not as accurate in assessing vascular stenosis or occlusions and distinction with atherosclerotic plaques that also show increased vascular uptake may be troublesome in older patients. Furthermore, a consensus agreement regarding [18]FDG-PET criteria of LV vasculitis is lacking. [18]FDG uptake equal to or greater than liver uptake on PET has been proposed as the best criterion of LV inflammation in GCA [84]. The vascular uptake in LV is also attenuated after three-day corticosteroid treatment but nevertheless, maintains an adequate sensitivity for diagnostic purposes. Notwithstanding, after ten days of treatment, sensitivity may diminish considerably (**Figure 4**) [85].

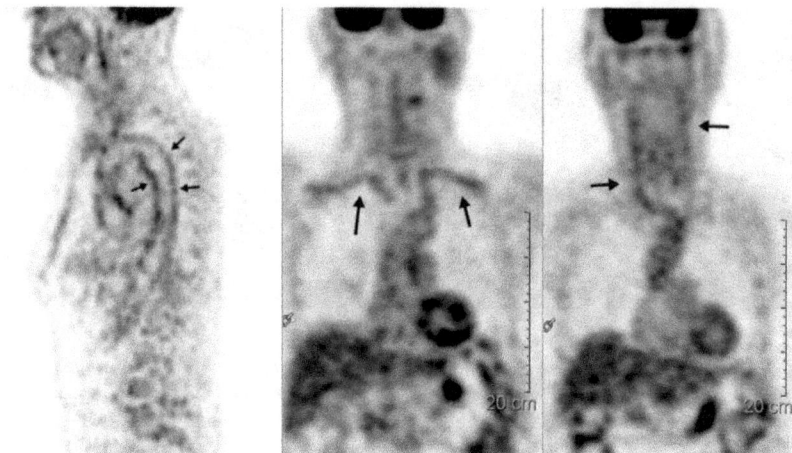

Figure 4.
^{18}FDG-PET scans of Large vessel GCA. Left panel shows aortitis with involvement of the thoracic and abdominal aorta. Central panel shouws inflammatory uptake of the ascendeing aorta and subclavian arteries. Reight panel reveals inflammatory uptake of the aorta and common carotid arteries. Arrows reveal areas of increased vascular ^{8}FDG uptake.

6. Treatment particularities

There are no studies specifically addressing the treatment of LV-GCA. As such, LV-GCA is currently managed in the same fashion of GCA. Corticosteroids remain the mainstay of treatment. Induction of remission should be started with 40-60 mg/day of prednisone equivalent to suppress systemic and vascular inflammation and prevent ischaemic complications such as blindness, and then followed by progressive tapering [2, 56, 86]. However, GCA relapses are frequent and corticosteroids account for significant complications. Therefore, adjunctive therapy should be considered in selected patients. Methotrexate (MTX) has been used as an adjunctive treatment with modest efficacy [87, 88]. TNF inhibitors have proven to be ineffective in GCA [89–91]. By contrast, the IL6-receptor blocker tocilizumab (TCZ) proved to be an effective and safe adjunctive therapy in GCA. Treatment with TCZ induced remission in over 50% of patients at 52 weeks, compared to less than 20% with placebo, and markedly reduced cumulative corticosteroid doses [92]. Recent results from real-life data corroborate the efficacy of TCZ shown in clinical trials [93].

There is some indirect evidence that LV vasculitis responds equally to standard treatment. This is corroborated by prospective imaging studies that show a decrease in LV inflammation over the course of treatment [76, 79, 85]. In a small study MTX was effective in corticosteroid-resistant LV-GCA [94]. However, it is widely accepted that patients with LV-GCA have a more relapsing disease course and receive higher doses of corticosteroids and more concomitant immunosuppressive therapy [7, 95].

In the GIACTA trial, 119 out of 251 patients included had evidence of LV vasculitis [96]. The outcomes measured did not include vascular imaging, and there is no sub-analysis directly aimed at patients with LV involvement. However, weekly TCZ was superior to biweekly TCZ or placebo in relapsing disease [92]. Being LV-GCA a more relapsing disease, it is possible that TCZ might be a preferred treatment option in this subgroup of patients [97].

Two other drugs have been studied in small GCA trials with data regarding LV-GCA. Ustekinumab, an IL-12/IL-23-blocking monoclonal antibody, was prospectively studied in 25 patients with refractory GCA, 10 of them with LV-GCA shown on CTA. Eight of these ten patients had multiple image assessments, and all of them showed improvement of wall thickening including four that had a complete resolution of the lesions [98]. However, in another prospective open-label trial with 13 patients with newly diagnosed or relapsing GCA, enrolment was prematurely closed due to lack of efficacy and high relapse rates [99]. Abatacept, an IgG1-CTLA4 fusion protein, was evaluated in a trial with 41 patients, (22% had LV vasculitis) and showed an improvement in relapse-free rate and duration of remission as compared to placebo [100]. Both these drugs need to be further evaluated in prospective and more extensive trials to further assess their efficacy.

Encouraging preliminary results were reported from a randomised controlled trial with mavrilumab, an anti-GM-CSF receptor α monoclonal antibody, which has shown sustained remission at week 26 in 83% of the patients, compared to 50% in the placebo group. These results were consistent across the different disease subgroups (final report is still pending) [101].

Another open question is whether current treatment significantly improves vascular remodelling and long-term LV-GCA complications such as aneurysms. The inhibition of both Jak1 and Jak2 may be a reasonable target to reduce the activation of the Th1 and Th17 pathways present in LV-GCA. Two Jak1 and Jak2 inhibitors are currently under investigation in clinical trials: baricitinib and upadacitinib [102, 103].

7. Complications and prognosis

Vascular complications of LV-GCA include the formation of arterial stenosis, occlusions and aneurysms [15, 16]. Involvement of the aorta commonly occurs as dilation or aneurysm, as aortic stenosis is unlikely. Stenosis presents as limb claudication, involving more commonly the superior extremities, although the involvement of the inferior extremity is also possible [7, 47]. GCA patients are at an increased risk of developing aortic aneurysms/dissection or large artery stenosis (**Figure 5**). While stenosis mostly occur during the first year, the incidence of aortic aneurysms/dissection increases over the five years following the GCA diagnosis [104].

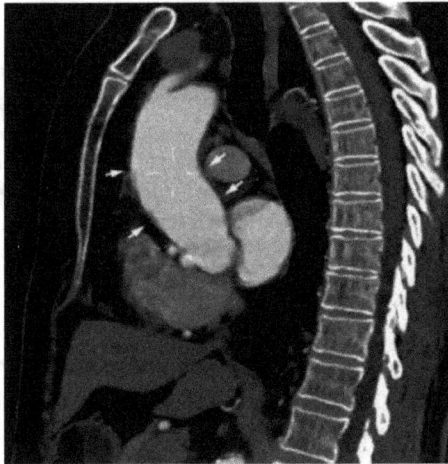

Figure 5.
Computed tomography angiography showing ascending aortic dilation in a patient with Giant Cell Arteritis.

In the long-term, 10–33% of the patients may develop aortic aneurysms/dissection and around 13% may develop large-artery stenosis [16, 104, 105].

Interestingly, aortic dilation is already present in 15% of the newly diagnosed GCA patients [12] with the thoracic aorta being the most commonly involved [105]. Aortic aneurysms are more frequently found among male patients with identified cardiovascular risk factors that include hypertension, dyslipidaemia and coronary artery disease [16, 17, 106]. It is unlikely that aortic aneurysms result from the persistent inflammatory activity as patients with aortic dilation/aneurysms were found to have lower serum acute-phase reactants and a lower relapse rate [17, 105]. However, increased [18]FDG uptake in the aorta on PET performed at the GCA diagnosis was associated with the subsequent development of aortic dilation [107, 108]. It is thus conceivable that a strong inflammatory response at the beginning of the disease followed by remodelling vascular factors and hemodynamic factors (like hypertension), may be more relevant to the development of aortic dilation and aneurysms than a continuous inflammatory process.

Despite all the possible complications, the overall prognosis of GCA is good, with a mortality rate similar to the general population [109]. However, GCA is responsible for a significant morbidity. Around 64% of the patients will have at least on relapse [52] and up to 86% of patients will develop at least on steroid related-complication [110]. Initially it would be thought that LV-GCA patients would not contribute to an increased morbidity as they have fewer ischaemic cranial events that classically have been responsible for the most relevant morbidity associated with GCA [10, 11].

However, LV-GCA patients have a more relapsing disease-course, have higher corticosteroid cumulative doses, and require additional immunosuppressive treatments [7, 95]. Moreover, patients with LV inflammation are at increased risk of developing large-artery stenosis and aortic arch syndrome [54, 105, 106]. In fact, when compared to the general population, survival is decreased in GCA patients with an aortic aneurysm/dissection [104], confirming the negative impact the involvement of large arteries has on both mortality and morbidity associated to GCA.

8. Conclusions

LV-GCA has been previously misregarded and underdiagnosed. However, there is consistent evidence confirming that large arteries are involved in around two-thirds of patients with GCA and one-third of patients with PMR. Classification criteria are inadequate for LV-GCA. A revision of the current criteria is required in the near future. LV-GCA presents a more relapsing-disease course and an increased risk of vascular complications, with LV inflammation being responsible for a considerable increment in the morbidity and mortality associated to this condition. This chapter emphasises the importance of carefully considering the large artery aspects in the management and treatment of patients with GCA.

Acknowledgements

We kindly thank Dr. Pedro Marques, from the Department of Radiology, Hospital Prof. Doutor Fernando Fonseca, for his collaboration with computed tomography image selection and editing.

We kindly thank Dr. Ângelo Ferreira Silva, from the Department of Nuclear Medicine, Champalimaud Foudation, for his collaboration with [18]FDG-PET image selection and editing.

Ultrasound images collected by the authors (Serôdio and Trindade) during the assessment of GCA patients with Siemens Acuson X300 equipment, VF13-5 probe, bandwidth 4,4-13,0 MHz.

Conflict of interest

The authors declare no conflict of interest.

Author details

João Fernandes Serôdio[1*], Miguel Trindade[1], Catarina Favas[1,2] and José Delgado Alves[1,2]

1 Department of Internal Medicine IV and Immune-Mediated Systemic Diseases Unit, Hospital Prof. Doutor Fernando Fonseca, Amadora, Portugal

2 Immune Response and Vascular Disease Unit, Chronic Diseases Research Centre CEDOC, Nova Medical School, Lisbon, Portugal

*Address all correspondence to: jserodio@campus.ul.pt

IntechOpen

References

[1] Jennette JC, Falk RJ, Bacon PA, et al. 2012 Revised International Chapel Hill consensus conference nomenclature of vasculitides. Arthritis Rheum. 2013; 65:1-11.

[2] Salvarani C, Pipitone N, Versari A, Hunder GG. Clinical features of polymyalgia rheumatica and giant cell arteritis. Nat Rev Rheumatol; 2012. 8;509-521.

[3] Gonzalez-Gay MA, Vazquez-Rodriguez TR, Lopez-Diaz MJ, et al. Epidemiology of giant cell arteritis and polymyalgia rheumatica. Arthritis Rheum; 2009. 61:1454-1461.

[4] Horton BT, Magath TB, Brown GE. An undescribed form of arteritis of the temporal vessels. Staff Meet Mayo Clin Proc. 1932;7:700-701.

[5] Gilmour JR. Giant-cell chronic arteritis. J Pathol Bacteriol. 1941;53(2):263-277.

[6] Hunder GG, Bloch DA, Michel BA, et al. The American College of Rheumatology 1990 criteria for the classification of giant cell arteritis. Arthritis Rheum. 1990;33(8): 1122-1128.

[7] Muratore F, Kermani TA, Crowson CS, et al. Large-vessel giant cell arteritis: A cohort study. Rheumatol. 2015; 54(3):463-470.

[8] Östberg G. Morphological changes in the large arteries in polymyalgia arteritica. Acta Med Scand Suppl. 1979;533:135-159.

[9] Ostberg G. Temporal arteritis in a large necropsy series. Ann Rheum Dis. 1971; 30:224-235.

[10] Schmidt WA, Seifert A, Gromnica-ihle E, et al. Ultrasound of proximal upper extremity arteries to increase the diagnostic yield in large-vessel giant cell arteritis. Rheumatology. 2008;47(1): 96-101.

[11] Aschwanden M, Kesten F, Stern M, et al. Vascular involvement in patients with giant cell arteritis determined by duplex sonography of 2x11 arterial regions. Ann Rheum Dis. 2010;69(7): 1356-1359.

[12] Prieto-González S, Arguis P, García-Martínez A, et al. Large vessel involvement in biopsy-proven giant cell arteritis: Prospective study in 40 newly diagnosed patients using CT angiography. Ann Rheum Dis. 2012;71(7):1170-1176.

[13] Narváez JA, Narváez JA, Nolla JM, et al. Giant cell arteritis and polymyalgia rheumatica: Usefulness of vascular magnetic resonance imaging studies in the diagnosis of aortitis. Rheumatology. 2005; 44(4):479-483.

[14] Blockmans D, De Ceuninck L, Vanderschueren S, et al. Repetitive 18F-fluorodeoxyglucose positron emission tomography in giant cell arteritis: A prospective study of 35 patients. Arthritis Care Res. 2006;55(1):131-137.

[15] Evans JM, O'Fallon WM, Hunder GG. Increased incidence of aortic aneurysm and dissection in giant cell (temporal) arteritis: A population-based study. Ann Intern Med. 1995;122(7):502-507.

[16] Nuenninghoff DM, Hunder GG, Christianson TJH, et al. Incidence and Predictors of Large-Artery Complication (Aortic Aneurysm, Aortic Dissection, and/or Large-Artery Stenosis) in Patients with Giant Cell Arteritis: A Population-Based Study over 50 Years. Arthritis Rheum. 2003;48(12):3522-3531.

[17] García-Martínez A, Hernández-Rodríguez J, Arguis P, et al. Development of aortic aneurysm/dilatation during the followup of patients with giant cell arteritis: A cross-sectional screening of fifty-four prospectively followed patients. Arthritis Care Res. 2008;59(3):422-430.

[18] Dejaco C, Duftner C, Buttgereit F, et al. The spectrum of giant cell arteritis and polymyalgia rheumatica: Revisiting the concept of the disease. Rheumatology. 2017; 56(4):506-515.

[19] Harky A, Fok M, Balmforth D, Bashir M. Pathogenesis of large vessel vasculitis: Implications for disease classification and future therapies. Vasc Med 2019; 24(1):79-88.

[20] Koster MJ, Warrington KJ. Classification of large vessel vasculitis: Can we separate giant cell arteritis from Takayasu arteritis? Press Medicale. 2017;46(7-8 Pt 2):e205–e213.

[21] Krupa WM, Dewan M, Jeon MS, et al. Trapping of misdirected dendritic cells in the granulomatous lesions of giant cell arteritis. Am J Pathol. 2002;161(5):1815-1823.

[22] Ma-Krupa W, Jeon MS, Spoerl S, et al. Activation of Arterial Wall Dendritic Cells and Breakdown of Self-tolerance in Giant Cell Arteritis. J Exp Med. 2004; 199(2):173-183.

[23] Dejaco C, Brouwer E, Mason JC, et al. Giant cell arteritis and polymyalgia rheumatica: Current challenges and opportunities. Nat Rev Rheumatol. 2017;13(10):578-592.

[24] Müller M, Briscoe J, Laxton C, et al. The protein tyrosine kinase JAK1 complements defects in interferon-α/β and -γ Signal transduction. Nature. 1993;366(6451):129-135.

[25] Espígol-Frigolé G, Corbera-Bellalta M, Planas-Rigol E, et al. Increased IL-17A expression in temporal artery lesions is a predictor of sustained response to glucocorticoid treatment in patients with giant-cell arteritis. Ann Rheum Dis. 2013;72(9):1481-1487.

[26] Hernández-Rodríguez J, Segarra M, Vilardell C, et al. Tissue production of pro-inflammatory cytokines (IL-1beta, TNFalpha and IL-6) correlates with the intensity of the systemic inflammatory response and with corticosteroid requirements in giant-cell arteritis. Rheumatology. 2004;43(3):294-301.

[27] Brack A, Rittner HL, Younge BR, et al. Glucocorticoid-mediated repression of cytokine gene transcription in human arteritis-SCID chimeras. J Clin Invest. 1997; 99(12):2842-2850.

[28] Kohlhuber, F. Rogers NC, Watling D, et al. A JAK1/JAK2 chimera can sustain alpha and gamma interferon responses. Mol Cell Biol. 1997; 17, 695-706.

[29] Cid MC, Prieto-Gonzalez S, Arguis P, et al. The spectrum of vascular involvement in giant-cell arteritis: Clinical consequences of detrimental vascular remodelling at different sites. APMIS Suppl; 2009. 27:10-20.

[30] Cid MC, Gandhi R, Corbera-Bellalta M, et al. THU0008 GM-CSF pathway signature identified in temporal artery biopsies of patients with giant cell arteritis. Ann Rheum Dis 2019;78:271-272.

[31] Rodríguez-Pla A, Bosch-Gil JA, Rosselló-Urgell J, et al. Metalloproteinase-2 and -9 in giant cell arteritis: Involvement in vascular remodeling. Circulation. 2005; 112(2):264-269.

[32] Weyand CM, Goronzy JJ. Immune mechanisms in medium and large-vessel vasculitis. Nat Rev Rheumatol; 2013. 9:731-740.

[33] Deng J, Younge BR, Olshen RA, et al. Th17 and Th1 T-cell responses in giant cell arteritis. Circulation. 2010 Feb;121(7):906-915.

[34] Visvanathan S, Rahman MU, Hoffman GS, et al. Tissue and serum markers of inflammation during the follow-up of patients with giant-cell arteritis--a prospective longitudinal study. Rheumatology. 2011; 50(11):2061-2070.

[35] Weyand CM, Hicok KC, Hunder GG, Goronzy JJ. Tissue cytokine patterns in patients with polymyalgia rheumatica and giant cell arteritis. Ann Intern Med. 1994;121(7):484-491.

[36] Deng J, Ma-Krupa W, Gewirtz AT, et al. Toll-like receptors 4 and 5 induce distinct types of vasculitis. Circ Res. 2009; 104(4):488-495.

[37] Pryshchep O, Ma-Krupa W, Younge BR, et al. Vessel-specific toll-like receptor profiles in human medium and large arteries. Circulation. 2008; 118(12):1276-1284.

[38] Graver JC, Boots AMH, Haacke EA, et al. Massive B-Cell Infiltration and Organization Into Artery Tertiary Lymphoid Organs in the Aorta of Large Vessel Giant Cell Arteritis. Front Immunol 2019; 10: 83.

[39] Gonzalez-Gay MA, Piñeiro A, Gomez-Gigirey A, et al. Influence of traditional risk factors of atherosclerosis in the development of severe ischemic complications in giant cell arteritis. Medicine. 2004; 83(6):342-347.

[40] Hernández-Rodríguez J, Segarra M, Vilardell C, et al. Elevated production of interleukin-6 is associated with a lower incidence of disease-related ischemic events in patients with giant-cell arteritis: Angiogenic activity of interleukin-6 as a potential protective mechanism. Circulation. 2003 ;107(19):2428-2434.

[41] Campbell BCV, De Silva DA, Macleod MR, et al. Ischaemic stroke. Nat Rev Dis Prim. 2019;5(1):70.

[42] Maksimowicz-Mckinnon K, Clark TM, Hoffman GS. Takayasu arteritis and giant cell arteritis: A spectrum within the same disease? Medicine. 2009; 88(4):221-226.

[43] McNulty M, Spiers P, McGovern E, Feelty L. Aging is associated with increased matrix metalloproteinase-2 activity in the human aorta. Am J Hypertens. 2005; 18(4):504-509.

[44] Ma Y, Chiao YA, Clark R, et al. Deriving a cardiac ageing signature to reveal MMP-9-dependent inflammatory signalling in senescence. Cardiovasc Res. 2015 Jun 1;106(3): 421-431.

[45] Najjar SS, Scuteri A, Lakatta EG. Arterial aging: Is it an immutable cardiovascular risk factor? Hypertension. 2005; 46:454-462.

[46] Saadoun D, Garrido M, Comarmond C, et al. Th1 and Th17 cytokines drive inflammation in Takayasu arteritis. Arthritis Rheumatol. 2015; 67(5):1353-1360.

[47] Kermani TA, Matteson EL, Hunder GG, Warrington KJ. Symptomatic lower extremity vasculitis in giant cell arteritis: A case series. J Rheumatol. 2009; 36(10):2277-2283.

[48] Diamantopoulos AP, Haugeberg G, Hetland H, et al. Diagnostic value of color doppler ultrasonography of temporal arteries and large vessels in giant cell arteritis: A consecutive case series. Arthritis Care Res. 2014; 66(1):113-119.

[49] Walter MA, Melzer RA, Schindler C, et al. The value of [18F] FDG-PET in the diagnosis of large-vessel vasculitis and the assessment of activity and extent of disease. Eur J Nucl

Med Mol Imaging. 2005
Jun;32(6):674-681.

[50] Salvarani C, Gabriel SE,
O'Fallon WM, Hunder GG.
Epidemiology of polymyalgia
rheumatica in Olmsted county,
Minnesota, 1970-1991. Arthritis Rheum.
1995;38(3):369-373.

[51] González-Gay MA, García-
Porrúa C, Vázquez-Caruncho M.
Polymyalgia rheumatica in biopsy
proven giant cell arteritis does not
constitute a different subset but differs
from isolated polymyalgia rheumatica.
J Rheumatol 1998; 25(9):1750-1755.

[52] Alba MA, García-Martínez A,
Prieto-González S, et al. Relapses in
patients with giant cell arteritis:
Prevalence, characteristics, and
associated clinical findings in a
longitudinally followed cohort of 106
patients. Medicine; 2014; 93(5):194-201.

[53] Blockmans D, Ceunick L,
Vanderschueren S, et al. Repetitive
18-fluorodeoxyglucose positron
emission tomography in isolated
polymyalgia rheumatica: a prospective
study in 35 patients. Rheumatology.
2007; 46:672-677

[54] Schmidt WA, Moll A, Seifert A,
et al. Prognosis of large-vessel giant cell
arteritis. Rheumatology. 2008;
47(9):1406-1408.

[55] Patil P, Williams M, Maw WW, et al.
Fast track pathway reduces sight loss in
giant cell arteritis: results of a
longitudinal observational cohort study.
Clin Exp Rheumatol. 2015 ;33(2):S-103.

[56] González-Gay MA, Blanco R,
Rodríguez-Valverde V, et al. Permanent
visual loss and cerebrovascular
accidents in giant cell arteritis:
Predictors and response to treatment.
Arthritis Rheum. 1998; 41(8):1497-1504.

[57] Diamantopoulos AP, Haugeberg G,
Lindland A, Myklebust G. The

fast-track ultrasound clinic for early
diagnosis of giant cell arteritis
significantly reduces permanent visual
impairment: Towards a more effective
strategy to improve clinical outcome in
giant cell arteritis? Rheumatology. 2016;
55(1):66-70.

[58] Ghinoi A, Pipitone N, Nicolini A,
et al. Large-vessel involvement in
recent-onset giant cell arteritis: A
case-control colour-doppler sonography
study. Rheumatology. 2012;
51(4):730-734.

[59] Monjo I, Fernández E, Peiteado D,
et al. OP0180 Diagnostic validity of
ultrasound including extra-cranial
arteries in Giant Cell Arteritis. Ann
Rheum Dis. 2020; 79-112.

[60] Onen F, Akkoc N. Epidemiology of
Takayasu arteritis. Press Medicale.
2017;46(7-8 Pt2):e197-203.

[61] Mason JC. Takayasu arteritis
advances in diagnosis and management.
Nat Rev Rheumatol. 2010;6(7):406-415.

[62] Ishikawa K. Diagnostic approach
and proposed criteria for the clinical
diagnosis of Takayasu's arteriopathy. J
Am Coll Cardiol. 1988;12(4):964-972.

[63] Grayson PC, Maksimowicz-
McKinnon K, Clark TM, et al.
Distribution of arterial lesions in
Takayasu's arteritis and giant cell
arteritis. Ann Rheum Dis. 2012
Aug;71(8):1329-1334.

[64] Kermani TA, Crowson CS,
Muratore F, et al. Extra-cranial giant cell
arteritis and Takayasu arteritis: How
similar are they? Semin Arthritis
Rheum. 2015; 44(6):724-728.

[65] Kerr GS, Hallahan CW, Giordano J,
et al. Takayasu arteritis. Ann Intern
Med. 1994 Jun 1;120(11):919-929.

[66] Esteban MJ, Font C, Hernández-
Rodríguez J, et al. Small-vessel vasculitis

surrounding a spared temporal artery: Clinical and pathologic findings in a series of twenty-eight patients. Arthritis Rheum. 2001;44(6):1387-1395.

[67] Chirinos JA, Tamariz LJ, Lopes G, et al. Large vessel involvement in ANCA-associated vasculitides: Report of a case and review of the literature. Clin Rheumatol. 2004; 23(2):152-159.

[68] Koster MJ, Matteson EL, Warrington KJ. Large-vessel giant cell arteritis: Diagnosis, monitoring and management. Rheumatology. 2018; 57(suppl_2):ii32–ii42.

[69] Gornik HL, Creager MA. Aortitis. Circulation. 2008; 117:3039-3051.

[70] Stone JH, Zen Y, Deshpande V. Mechanisms of disease: IgG4-related disease. N Engl J Med. 2012;366(6):539-551.

[71] Haroche J, Arnaud L, Amoura Z. Erdheim-chester disease. Current Opinion in Rheumatology. Curr Opin Rheumatol. 2012; 24:53-59.

[72] Palazzi C, Salvarani C, D'Angelo S, Olivieri I. Aortitis and periaortitis in ankylosing spondylitis. Joint Bone Spine. 2011; 78:451-455.

[73] Luqmani R, Lee E, Singh S, et al. The role of ultrasound compared to biopsy of temporal arteries in the diagnosis and treatment of giant cell arteritis (TABUL): A diagnostic accuracy and cost-effectiveness study. Health Technol Assess. 2016; 20(90):1-270.

[74] Schmidt WA, Kraft HE, Vorpahl K,et al. Color Duplex Ultrasonography in the Diagnosis of Temporal Arteritis. N Engl J Med. 1997; 337(19):1336-1342.

[75] Schäfer VS, Juche A, Ramiro S, et al. Ultrasound cut-off values for intima-media thickness of temporal, facial and axillary arteries in giant cell arteritis. Rheumatology. 2017; 56(9):1479-1483.

[76] De Miguel E, Roxo A, Castillo C, et al. The utility and sensitivity of colour Doppler ultrasound in monitoring changes in giant cell arteritis. Clin Exp Rheumatol. 2012; 30(1Suppl 70):S34-S38.

[77] Agard C, Barrier JH, Dupas B, et al. Aortic involvement in recent-onset giant cell (temporal) arteritis: A case-control prospective study using helical aortic computed tomodensitometric scan. Arthritis Care Res. 2008; 59(5):670-676.

[78] Hervé F, Choussy V, Janvresse A, et al. Aortic involvement in giant cell arteritis. A prospective follow-up of 11 patients using computed tomography. Rev Med Interne. 2006; 27(3):196-202.

[79] Prieto-González S, García-Martínez A, Tavera-Bahillo I, et al. Effect of glucocorticoid treatment on computed tomography angiography detected large-vessel inflammation in giant-cell arteritis. A prospective, longitudinal study. Medicine. 2015; 94(5):e486.

[80] Prieto-González S, Arguis P, Cid MC. Imaging in systemic vasculitis. Curr Opin Rheumatol. 2015; 27:53-62.

[81] Klink T, Geiger J, Both M, et al. Giant cell arteritis: Diagnostic accuracy of mr imaging of superficial cranial arteries in initial diagnosis-results from a multicenter trial. Radiology 2014;273(3):844-582.

[82] Quinn KA, Ahlman MA, Malayeri AA, et al. Comparison of magnetic resonance angiography and 18 F-fluorodeoxyglucose positron emission tomography in large-vessel vasculitis. Ann Rheum Dis. 2018; 77(8):1166-1172.

[83] Lariviere D, Benali K, Coustet B, et al. Positron emission tomography and computed tomography angiography for

the diagnosis of giant cell arteritis: A real-life prospective study. Medicine. 2016; 96(30):e4146.

[84] Soussan M, Nicolas P, Schramm C, et al. Management of large-vessel vasculitis: a systematic literature reviwe and meta-analysis with FDG-PET. Medicine. 2015; 94(14):e622

[85] Nielsen BD, Gormsen LC, Hansen IT, et al. Three days of high-dose glucocorticoid treatment attenuates large-vessel 18F-FDG uptake in large-vessel giant cell arteritis but with a limited impact on diagnostic accuracy. Eur J Nucl Med Mol Imaging. 2018; 45(7):1119-1128.

[86] Hellmich B, Agueda A, Monti S, et al. 2018 Update of the EULAR recommendations for the management of large vessel vasculitis. Ann Rheum Dis. 2020;79(1):19-30.

[87] Hoffman GS, Cid MC, Hellmann DB, et al. A multicenter, randomized, double-blind, placebo-controlled trial of adjuvant methotrexate treatment for giant cell arteritis. Arthritis Rheum. 2002;46(5):1309-1318.

[88] Jover JA, Hernández-García C, Morado IC, et al. Combined treatment of giant-cell arteritis with methotrexate and prednisone: A randomized, double-blind, placebo-controlled trial. Ann Intern Med. 2001;134(2):106-114.

[89] Hoffman GS, Cid MC, Rendt-Zagar KE, et al. Infliximab for maintenance of glucocorticosteroid-induced remission of giant cell arteritis a randomized trial. Ann Intern Med. 2007;146(9):621-630.

[90] Martínez-Taboada VM, Rodríguez-Valverde V, Carreño L, et al. A double-blind placebo controlled trial of etanercept in patients with giant cell arteritis and corticosteroid side effects. Ann Rheum Dis. 2008;67(5):625-630.

[91] Seror R, Baron G, Hachulla E, et al. Adalimumab for steroid sparing in patients with giant-cell arteritis: Results of a multicentre randomised controlled trial. Ann Rheum Dis. 2014;73(12):2074-2081.

[92] Stone JH, Tuckwell K, Dimonaco S, et al. Trial of Tocilizumab in Giant-Cell Arteritis. N Engl J Med. 2017;377(4): 317-328.

[93] Calderón-Goercke M, Castañeda S, Aldasoro V, et al. Tocilizumab in giant cell arteritis: differences between the GiACTA trial and a multicentre series of patients from the clinical practice. Clin Exp Rheumatol. 2020;38(2):112-119.

[94] Camellino, D; Morbelli S, Sambuceti GCM. Methotrexate treatment of polymyalgia rheumatica/giant cell arteritis associated large vessel vasculitis. Clin Exp Rheumatol. 2010;28:288-289.

[95] Muratore F, Bolardi L, Restuccia G, et al. Relapses and long-term remission in large vessel giant cell arteritis in northern Italy: Characteristics and predictors in a long-term follow-up study. Sem Arthritis Rheum. 2020; 50(4):549-558.

[96] Tuckwell K, Collinson N, Klearman M, et al. FRI0377 Classification Criteria for Giant Cell Arteritis: Data from Giacta Informing The Need for Revision. Ann Rheum Dis 2016;75:571.

[97] Leuchten N, Aringer M. Tocilizumab in the treatment of giant cell arteritis. Immunotherapy. 2018;10(6):465-472.

[98] Conway R, O'Neill L, O'Flynn E, et al. Ustekinumab for the treatment of refractory giant cell arteritis. Ann Rheum Dis. 2016; 75:1578-1579.

[99] Matza MA, Fernandes AD, Stone JH, Unizony SH. Ustekinumab for

the Treatment of Giant Cell Arteritis. Arthritis Care Res. 2020; doi: 10.1002/acr.24378.

[100] Langford CA, Cuthbertson D, Ytterberg SR, et al. A Randomized, Double-Blind Trial of Abatacept (CTLA-4Ig) for the Treatment of Giant Cell Arteritis. Arthritis Rheumatol. 2017; 69(4):837-845.

[101] Cid M, Unizony S, Pupim L, et al. Mavrilimumab (anti GM-CSF Receptor α Monoclonal Antibody) Reduces Time to Flare and Increases Sustained Remission in a Phase 2 Trial of Patients with Giant Cell Arteritis. Arthritis Rheumatol. 2020;72(Suppl 10).

[102] Baricitinib in Relapsing Giant Cell Arteritis C.incialTrials.gov: clinicaltrials.gov/ct2/show/NCT03026504

[103] A Study to Evaluate the Safety and Efficacy of Upadacitinib in Participants With Giant Cell Arteritis. ClinicalTrials.gov:clinicaltrials.gov/ct2/show/NCT03725202

[104] Kermani TA, Warrington KJ, Crowson CS, et al. Large-vessel involvement in giant cell arteritis: A population-based cohort study of the incidence-trends and prognosis. Ann Rheum Dis. 2013;72(12):1989-1994.

[105] García-Martínez A, Arguis P, et al. Prospective long term follow-up of a cohort of patients with giant cell arteritis screened for Aortic structural damage (aneurysm or dilatation). Ann Rheum Dis. 2014;73(10):1826-1832.

[106] Gonzalez-Gay MA, Garcia-Porrua C, et al. Aortic aneurysm and dissection in patients with biopsy-proven giant cell arteritis from northwestern Spain: A population-based study. Medicine. 2004;83(6):335-341.

[107] Blockmans D, Coudyzer W, Vanderschueren S, et al. Relationship between fluorodeoxyglucose uptake in the large vessels and late aortic diameter in giant cell arteritis. Rheumatology. 2008;47(8):1179-1184.

[108] De Boysson H, Liozon E, Lambert M, Parienti JJ, Artigues N, Geffray L, et al. 18 F-fluorodeoxyglucose positron emission tomography and the risk of subsequent aortic complications in giant-cell arteritis. Medicine. 2016;95(26):e3851.

[109] Matteson EL, Gold KN, Bloch DA, Hunder GG. Long-term survival of patients with giant cell arteritis in the American College of Rheumatology giant cell arteritis classification criteria cohort. Am J Med. 1996;100(2):193-196.

[110] Proven A, Gabriel SE, Orces C, et al. Glucocorticoid Therapy in Giant Cell Arteritis: Duration and Adverse Outcomes. Arthritis Care Res. 2003;49(5):703-708.

Chapter 4

Medical Image Processing and Analysis Techniques for Detecting Giant Cell Arteritis

Radwan Qasrawi, Diala Abu Al-Halawa, Omar Daraghmeh, Mohammad Hjouj and Rania Abu Seir

Abstract

Medical image segmentation and classification algorithms are commonly used in clinical applications. Several automatic and semiautomatic segmentation methods were used for extracting veins and arteries on transverse and longitudinal medical images. Recently, the use of medical image processing and analysis tools improved giant cell arteries (GCA) detection and diagnosis using patient specific medical imaging. In this chapter, we proposed several image processing and analysis algorithms for detecting and quantifying the GCA from patient medical images. The chapter introduced the connected threshold and region growing segmentation approaches on two case studies with temporal arteritis using ultrasound (US) and magnetic resonance imaging (MRI) imaging modalities extracted from the Radiopedia Dataset. The GCA detection procedure was developed using the 3D Slicer Medical Imaging Interaction software as a fast prototyping open-source framework. GCA detection passes through two main procedures: The pre-processing phase, in which we improve and enhances the quality of an image after removing the noise, irrelevant and unwanted parts of the scanned image by the use of filtering techniques, and contrast enhancement methods; and the processing phase which includes all the steps of processing, which are used for identification, segmentation, measurement, and quantification of GCA. The semi-automatic interaction is involved in the entire segmentation process for finding the segmentation parameters. The results of the two case studies show that the proposed approach managed to detect and quantify the GCA region of interest. Hence, the proposed algorithm is efficient to perform complete, and accurate extraction of temporal arteries. The proposed semi-automatic segmentation method can be used for studies focusing on three-dimensional visualization and volumetric quantification of Giant Cell Arteritis.

Keywords: Giant Cell Arteritis, Enhancement, Detection and Classification, Segmentation

1. Introduction

Giant cell arteritis (GCA), also called temporal arteritis or cranial arteritis is a systemic inflammation of medium to large-sized vessels [1]. The cause of the disease is currently unknown; however, autoimmunity is one hypothesis [2].

GCA most commonly occurs in females (female to male ratio 2-4:1) over the age of 50 years [3]. Temporal artery involvement classically presents with sudden onset of severe headache associated with inflammatory and ischemic symptoms; [1] however, GCA may involve other large-sized arteries, namely the aorta, subclavian, iliac, ophthalmic, occipital, and vertebral arteries, which have different presentation and may be involved independently from the cranial arteries [4].

Left untreated, GCA can lead to permanent visual loss and various systemic complications; therefore, there is a need for effective diagnosis. The American College of Rheumatology proposed criteria for the diagnosis of GCA [5]. The diagnosis mainly relies on clinical presentation, inflammatory markers (typically high erythrocyte sedimentation rate (ESR)), and usually histological confirmation by temporal artery biopsy. Temporal artery biopsy has been the standard test to confirm the diagnosis of GCA, which although highly specific, is considered invasive and lacks sensitivity [2, 6, 7]. Consequently, diagnosis of GCA often relies on the combination of clinical symptoms, serum inflammatory markers, and radiological imaging.

2. Diagnosis of GCA by radiological imaging

The role of radiological imaging is becoming increasingly important in the diagnosis and follow-up of GCA. Generally, the different radiological imaging modalities visualize different aspects of the involved vessel wall thickening and luminal stenosis. The first line imaging modality, especially for cranial GCA is color duplex sonography (CDS) [4, 8, 9]. CDS assesses vascular wall anatomy and luminal lining and diameter. A characteristic finding of GCA on CDS is the (halo) sign, which is homogenous, hypoechogenic circumferential vessel wall thickening. Another finding is the lack of compressibility of the artery manifested by the application of transducer-imposed pressure on the temporal arteries (compression sign) [4, 8]. The (halo) sign has a sensitivity ranging from 55 to 100% and specificity of 78 to 100% in the diagnosis of temporal arteritis [8]. The wide range of sensitivity may be attributed to operator experience and arterial involvement. A systematic review published in 2016 discussed the use of the different imaging modalities in the diagnosis and follow-up of GCA [10]. The review findings suggest that CDS is an easy, cost-effective diagnostic imaging tool for the evaluation of cranial vessels, as well as the carotid, subclavian, axillary, and brachial vessels. The reliability of the unilateral halo sign is debatable; however, the presence of a bilateral (halo) sign discards the need for temporal artery biopsy. Many studies have compared ultrasound (US) imaging versus temporal artery biopsy in the evaluation of GCA [11–15]. In a prospective cohort study published in 2019, Zou *et al.* discussed the results of clinical examination following the US versus biopsy of the temporal artery biopsy directly, considering MRI as a reference diagnostic data. The study included 980 patients with a mean age of 61.12 ± 6.56 years who complained of at least one symptom consistent with GCA but have not been diagnosed or treated with glucocorticoids [11, 14]. US and MRI imaging included bilateral temporal arteries, axillary arteries, and their branches. The study concluded that the clinical examination following US detection of GCA had high accuracy and a lower risk of overdiagnosis and unnecessary glucocorticoid treatment of low to medium risk GCA [2]. Moreover, there was a higher number of false-negative diagnoses reported by temporal artery biopsy. These results are consistent with other studies like the TABUL study [1].

Other important noninvasive imaging modalities are contrast-enhanced computed tomography (CT) scan and CT angiography (CTA). Both scans visualize cranial and extracranial arteries, the aorta for example, and can visualize associated complications [16, 17]. On CT, the diseased vessel wall appears edematous with concentric enlargement and usually shows late contrast enhancement. CTA on the other hand is better for visualization of the luminal vascular pathology. Both modalities are excellent for the diagnosis of GCA when the involvement of a large-sized vessel other than the temporal artery is suspected. However, there is a scarcity of data on the use of CT/CTA in the diagnosis of GCA. Berthod *et al.* discussed in a case–control study CT imaging of the aorta in suspected GCA, which included 174 participants (64 with GCA, 43 with polymyalgia rheumatica, and 67 controls) [18]. The study results showed that using CT in the evaluation of the aorta is diagnostic of GCA which is morphologically different that atheromatous lesions. The study set an aortic wall thickness of ≥ 2.2 mm as pathological and indicative of GCA.

Additionally, magnetic resonance imaging (MRI) and MR-angiography (MRA) have a prominent role in the diagnosis of GCA. The t2 weighted MRI images show a hyperintense rim at the edematous segment of the vessel wall. Moreover, t1 weighted images depict mural thickening and contrast enhancement. MRA, as CTA, better visualizes irregular luminal lining and can assess the extent of arterial wall damage and the effectiveness of treatment [8]. The use of MRI in the clinical setting is available; however, its diagnostic accuracy is still indefinite as the available literature has approached this issue differently. A systematic literature review and meta-analysis discussed the diagnostic accuracy of MRI imaging of the temporal and occipital arteries. They reviewed six studies with 509 patients that used either clinical diagnosis or temporal artery biopsy as the reference standard. They found that when the clinical diagnosis was used as the reference standard, MRI had a lower pooled sensitivity and specificity (73%, 88%) than that of the US (77% and 96%, respectively). However, when compared with temporal artery biopsy, MRI had a higher sensitivity (93% vs. 70%) and a similar specificity to sonography (81% vs. 84%). Thus, they advised that both modalities have good diagnostic accuracy of superficial temporal arteries GCA [17].

Furthermore, fluoro-D-glucose integrated with computed tomography (FDG-PET/CT) is also currently used in the diagnosis of large-sized vascular wall inflammation. This modality shows the increased uptake of glucose by the inflammatory cells lining the vessel wall [19].

The choice of image processing technique depends on the available imaging modality and the level of expertise in the clinical setting, taking on consideration the risks of radiation or contrast exposure, in contrast to the benefit of timely and accurate diagnosis of GCA versus the overdiagnosis and overtreatment of GCA based on conventional diagnostic criteria. The European League Against Rheumatism (EULAR) has issued recommendations on the use of different imaging modalities in the evaluation of large vessel vasculitis [20]. However, currently, there is no clearly defined protocol for imaging in suspected GCA; yet, there is increasing attention over the advantages and disadvantages of using each imaging modality in accordance with the clinical presentation.

3. GCA image processing and analysis

Recently, the use of medical image processing and analysis tools improved GCA detection and diagnosis using medical imaging. These tools provide physicians with semi-automatic detection and quantification of suspected regions of interest and enhance GCA diagnosis.

Medical imaging processing refers to the process of digital imaging by using computer software. This process includes several types of techniques and operations such as image enhancement, segmentation, registration, and visualization [21].

The rapid advancement of image processing and analysis improved the medical care process in clinical applications.

The current advances in medical imaging made in medical fields such as imaging modalities, diagnostics, and treatment applications are designed on digital imaging technology processing and analysis. Medical image processing has been recognized as a source of innovation in the advanced medical care process including medical informatics, artificial intelligence, and bioinformatics. Recently, many libraries, tools, and software products can process and manipulate images from different modalities (CT, MRI, US, PET) and are available for clinical application and research purposes [22].

Medical image segmentation and classification algorithms are commonly used in clinical applications. Several automatic and semiautomatic segmentation methods were used for extracting veins and arteries on transverse and longitudinal medical images [23]. The deformable contour model, connected threshold, fast marching method, and many other methods were used for extracting the arteries from US images. Other studies reported the application of region growing, diffusion-based filter, edge detection combined with morphology methods, and Hough transforms [12, 23, 24]. In this chapter, we proposed several image processing and analysis algorithms for detecting and quantifying the GCA from patient medical images. The chapter introduced the connected threshold segmentation approach on two case studies for temporal arteritis using US and MRI imaging modalities extracted from the Radiopedia Dataset [12].

4. GCA image processing and analysis software

The GCA detection procedure was developed using the 3D Slicer Medical Imaging Interaction software as a fast prototyping open-source framework [25]. The 3D slicer is a free open-source software system providing extendibility by plug-ins development that interacts with the application core. It is an open-source software platform for medical image informatics, image processing, and three-dimensional visualization. Built over two decades through support from the National Institutes of Health and a worldwide developer community, Slicer brings free, powerful cross-platform processing tools to physicians, researchers, and the general public.

The main focus of the 3D slicer is to enable the creation of highly interactive medical imaging software applications; it integrates different tools for medical imaging, computational modeling, computer graphics, deep learning, and numerical modeling for building applications with complex interaction mechanisms. It also provides a graphical user interface, multiple consistent views for the same data, 3D rendering, data retrieval, hierarchical organization for data objects, advanced visualization of multi-modal imaging, and support for 3D + t data.

3D slicer is an object-oriented cross-platform library implemented in C++ that supports Windows, Linux, and macOS. It integrates and extends widely-used open-source C++ libraries which are the Visualization Toolkit (VTK) and the Insight Toolkit (ITK), both supported by Kitware Inc. The ITK is an open-source, cross-platform library that provides an extensive suite of software algorithms for image analysis, it builds a set of fundamental algorithms especially for segmentation and registration. While the VTK supports a wide variety of visualization algorithms and advanced modeling techniques.

In addition to ITK and VTK, third-party packages can be integrated and used with MITK, such as the DICOM Toolkit (DCMTK, supported by Offis in Germany), and other commonly used C++ libraries (Boost, Qt, OpenCV among others). The software includes numerous modules, extensions, datasets, pull requests, patches, issues report, suggestions—is made possible by users, developers, contributors, and commercial partners around the world. This development is funded by various grants and agencies [26].

5. Giant cell arteritis detection using medical image processing and analysis

Medical imaging is a commonly used method for detecting GCA and the diagnosis of arteries related diseases. Nowadays, medical image processing and analysis methods are used to facilitate the identification of the boundaries of internal organs from medical images and thus enhance the diagnostics of specific abnormalities. Patients with GCA may be indicated for medical imaging examination for initial diagnosing or monitoring of the disease activities.

GCA detection can be defined as the procedure in which the GCA region of interest can be detected and identified from medical images. In clinical application, the GCA diagnostic planning is defined as the process in which it is planned, using the computer system, where the GCA disease can be detected and quantified.

GCA detection passes through two main procedures: the pre-processing phase and the processing and analysis phase. The pre-processing phase improves and enhances the quality of an image after removing the noise, irrelevant and unwanted parts of the scanned image. The enhancement of image quality is obtained by the use of filtering techniques, removal of noise, and contrast enhancement methods. The processing phase includes all the steps of processing, which are used for identification, segmentation, measurement, and quantification of GCA.

GCA segmentation is composed of a series of image processing algorithms that depend on the medical image type and quality. The core image processing algorithms include:

a. The image enhancement and denoising algorithms:

1. Gaussian Blur Module and Gaussian Blur Batch Make Module: these modules convolve the image with a Gaussian kernel wherein the Gaussian has a standard deviation specified by the user (GUI field "sigma") and the kernel width in each dimension is 6 times the standard deviation of the Gaussian.

2. The Median Image Filter is commonly used as a robust approach for noise reduction. This filter is particularly efficient against 'salt-and-pepper' noise. In other words, it is robust to the presence of gray-level outliers. Median Image Filter computes the value of each output pixel as the statistical median of the neighborhood of values around the corresponding input pixel.

3. Image editing tools include cropping, adding and subtracting, cutting, change the directions and orientations.

b. Image processing and analysis that includes:

1. Threshold selection based on pixel intensity histogram analysis.

2. Image segmentation with the selected threshold result and the use of an interactive segmentation tool that allows physicians to edit, and modify the segmented region as requested.

c. Region of interest post-processing that includes surface or volume reconstruction, measurements, deformation, and simplifications for clinical application. The measurements include the calculation of ROI area, volume, distances from organs, and other basic measurements and statistics (Mean, median, SD...etc).

The proposed method for detecting the GCA is shown in **Figure 1**. The image enhancement and the segmentation based on the threshold method are calculated from 2D MRI and US image slices. The US image shows the left temporal artery, and the MRI shows the right temporal right artery segmentation.

This approach of segmentation allows the semi-automatic detection of the outlines of the artery in the enhanced medical image. The methods of segmentation by the threshold, region growing, and interactive segmentation is commonly used in the literature. In this chapter, we tested the methods on two case studies using semi-automatic methods for detecting the GCA.

The semi-automatic segmentation is done by studying the histogram and the threshold analysis of the 2D US and MRI images. The histogram analysis is used to identify the pixel densities of all areas of interest. In this study, we assumed that there are differences calcification density distribution between the blood,

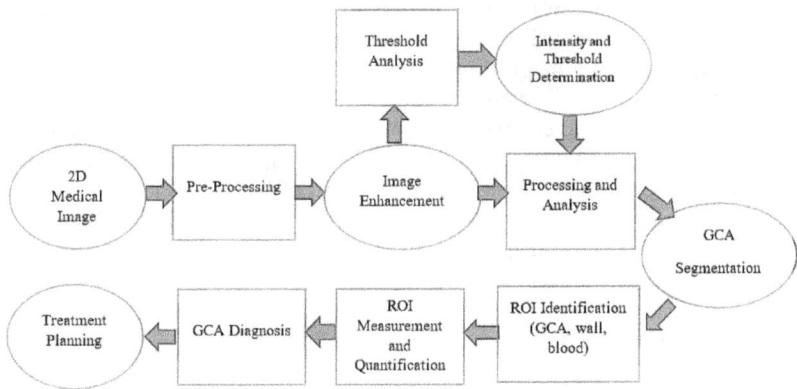

Figure 1.
The flow chart GCA detection method.

US image Case Study					
	Volume [cm³]	Threshold (Pixel Densities)	Diameter [mm]	Surface area [mm²]	Roundness
Temporal Artery Wall	3.29	−85 − −25.3	181	8622.2	0.12
GCA Wall Thickening	0.73	−87− −32.9	160	1989.5	0.25
MRI Image Case Study					
Temporal Artery Wall	2.31	−376 − −127.6	201	4618.9	0.18
GCA Wall Thickening	0.28	−400 − −157.4	88	594.3	0.35

Table 1.
The US and MRI histogram and statistical analysis.

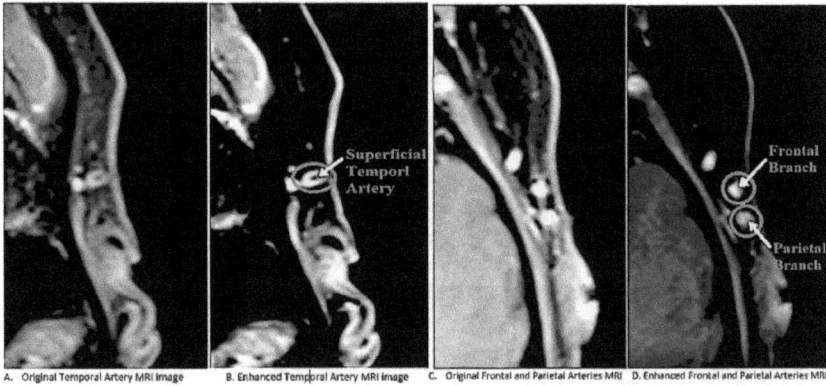

Figure 2.
Pre-processing filters and algorithms for the enhancement of MRI image of a 50 years old female patient.

artery wall, and the GCA region since the density of the GCA region is often lower than the blood and the normal wall densities. The image histogram analysis is summarized in **Table 1**. The temporal artery wall and the GCA wall thickening diameters were calculated in both images, the results in **Table 1** show an increase in the artery wall in both cases (160 mm and 88 mm). Furthermore, the GCA artery wall roundness was higher than the normal artery roundness in both cases (0.25 mm and 0.35 mm), respectively. The pixel density threshold analysis shows that there are few differences between the normal and GCA regions as indicated in **Table 1**.

In the pre-processing phase, various filtering and thresholding algorithms are applied successively to obtain the artery contour and boundary. This contour is separated and segmented into three contours (regions): the artery wall, the blood, and the abnormal region (GCA). Results in **Figure 2** show the two cases before and after image pre-processing.

The segmented regions were quantified and measured using the 3D slicer measurement and quantification tools.

6. Giant cell arteriti's case studies

In this chapter, two case studies were conducted to assess the connected threshold and region growing segmentation algorithms as a semi-automatic detection and quantification of temporal arteritis on US and MRA images. The histogram threshold analysis was performed to analyze and study the pixel distribution in both mages. Otsu's method was used to divide the images into two parts, namely; foreground and background regions. To segment the temporal artery, we performed the threshold segmentation algorithm on the foreground region by comparing two different statistical distributions. The semi-automatically segmented regions were compared with manually segmented regions. The segmentations were validated by experts and the different similarity metrics were used to identify the variations in segmentation.

6.1 US case study

In the clinical application, the temporal artery characteristics can be found and detected using US images. GCA detection compared to the normal artery is

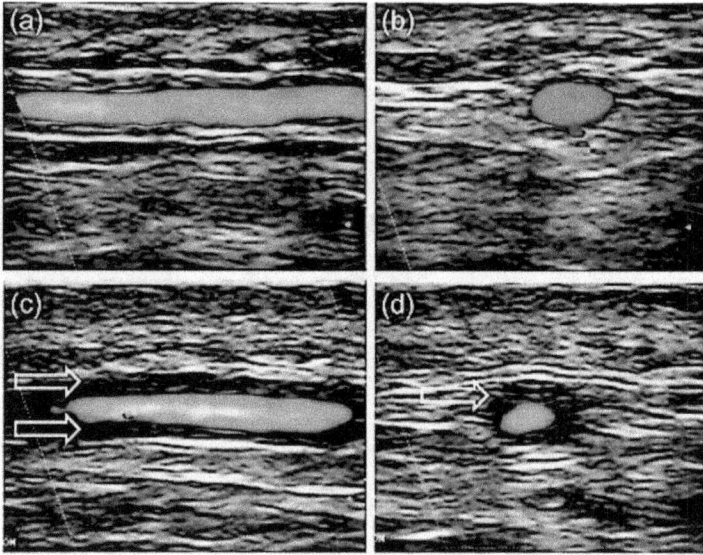

Figure 3.
Color doppler ultrasound showing longitudinal (a) and transverse (b) views of normal temporal artery and acute temporal arteritis. (c, d) The arrows indicate the vasculitis wall swelling [27].

shown in **Figure 3** [27]. The data in **Figure 3(a)** and **(b)** show the longitudinal and transverse views of normal temporal artery and acute temporal arteritis in **Figure 2(c)** and **(d)** of an adult women aged 45 years old. As seen in **Figure 2**, the arrows indicate the vasculitis wall swelling. The ultrasonography features showed a hypoechogenic halo of the temporal artery in longitudinal (left) and transverse (right) view. The data show that the normal artery diameter is 0.3-1 mm and the temporal artery diameter is 1-2 mm.

In our proposed method, the US image data of a 40 years old female patient with a visible thickening of the left temporal artery that causes a chronic left temporal headache was used to test our segmentation method. [Radiopaedia. org/GCA case studies] The data is validated by comparing the artery wall segmentation results with the manual ones from experts. The typical US image used in this chapter is shown in **Figure 4(a)** and **(b)**. **Figure 4(a)** shows a longitudinal view of GCA with wall thickness on the lower side of the temporal artery. **Figure 4(b)** shows the results of segmented regions using the threshold segmentation. The area in yellow represents the wall segment, the red indicates the blood segment while the green area represents the GCA region of interest. The temporal artery has been well-segmented and the clinical characteristics have been identified and documented. The results show the diameters of the lumen, wall, and the blood flows velocity at the region of interest along with the superficial temporal artery. The diameter of the artery wall was significantly thicker than the normal artery. The GCA region of interest diameter was 1.6 mm with an area of 19.9 cm^2.

6.2 MRI case study

The MRI case study represents a patient of a 50-year-old female with clinical suspicion of temporal arteritis, the left temporal artery and its frontal and parietal branches show significant wall thickening [12].

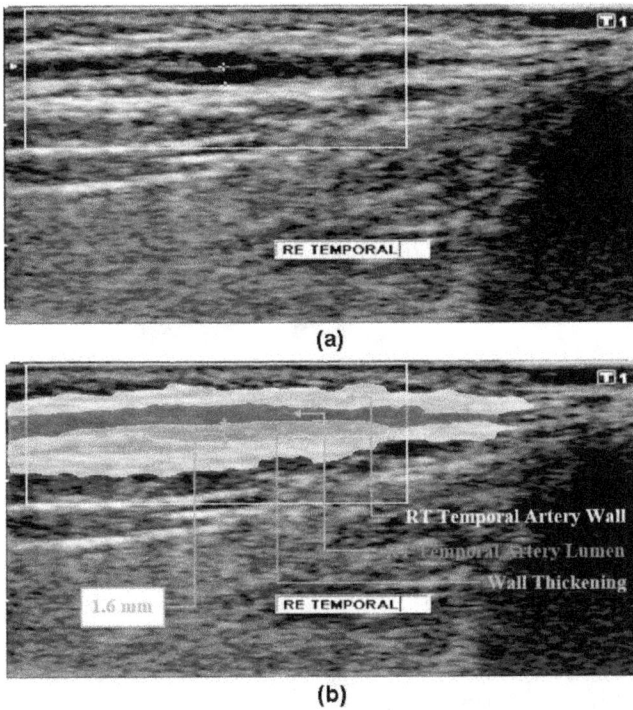

Figure 4.
The left temporal artery of 40 years female patient, (a) shows the temporal artery before segmentation, (b) the threshold segmentation of GCA region of interest [12].

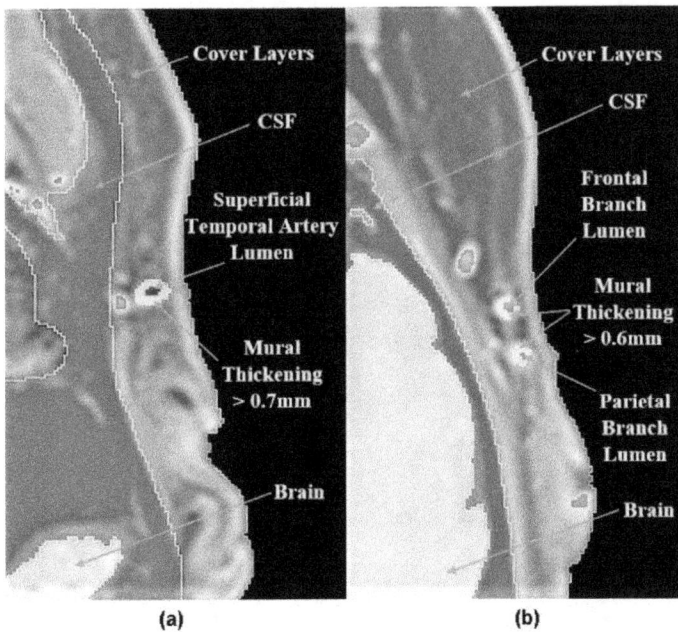

Figure 5.
The left temporal artery of 50 years female patient, (a) shows the temporal artery before segmentation, (b) the threshold segmentation of GCA region of interest [12].

Prominent mural enhancement is identified in these arteries when compared to the contralateral side. The contralateral temporal artery and its branches show a normal appearance.

The high-resolution MRI imaging of the superficial temporal artery is shown in **Figure 5(a)** and **(b)**. The arrow in **Figure 5(a)** shows the position of the abnormal temporal arteries. The images in **Figure 5(b)** show the frontal branch and the parietal branch after image pre-processing and enhancement. The region growing segmentation of the region of interest in both images shows the GCA regions. The average superficial temporal artery wall thickness was 0.71 mm. According to the literature mural thickening > 0.5 mm was considered as a sign of mural inflammation [28].

7. Conclusion

In this chapter, we discussed the use of medical image processing and analysis in detecting and quantification of GCA. We discussed a semi-automated segmentation of temporal arteries from 2D temporal artery US and MRI images using image processing and analysis algorithms. These algorithms depend on various image processing algorithms, including image enhancement, noise reduction, pixel densities histogram analysis, and statistical analysis tools. First, the Gaussian filters and noise reduction algorithms are applied to enhance the temporal artery structures, which effectively enhances the temporal artery contrast, because the shape information of the blood flow is considered. Afterward, seed points are detected automatically through threshold pre-processing operation. Based on the set of seed points and threshold analysis, region growing is applied, which grows in the target region. Then, the temporal artery region is extracted by connected threshold and region growing approaches, which are capable of segmenting the artery due to the pixel intensity thresholds and the seed point approach. Three regions of interest were extracted, the temporal artery wall, the blood flow, and the GCA region. Then the statistical and measurement tools are used to quantify the diameters, area, and volume of the GCA regions, and to detect and identify the size and location of the GCA region. The semi-automatic interaction is involved in the entire segmentation process for finding the segmentation parameters. Hence, the proposed algorithm is efficient to perform complete, and accurate extraction of temporal arteries. The proposed semi-automatic segmentation method can be used for studies focusing on three-dimensional visualization and volumetric quantification of Giant Cell Arteritis.

Author details

Radwan Qasrawi[1*], Diala Abu Al-Halawa[2], Omar Daraghmeh[3], Mohammad Hjouj[3] and Rania Abu Seir[3]

1 Faculty of Science and Technology, Al-Quds University, Palestine

2 Faculty of Medicine, Al-Quds University, Palestine

3 Faculty of Health Professions, Al-Quds University, Palestine

*Address all correspondence to: radwan@staff.alquds.edu

IntechOpen

References

[1] M. A. Ameer, R. J. Peterfy, P. Bansal, and B. Khazaeni, "Temporal Arteritis," *StatPearls [Internet]*, 2020.

[2] H. S. Lyons, V. Quick, A. J. Sinclair, S. Nagaraju, and S. P. Mollan, "A new era for giant cell arteritis," *Eye*, vol. 34, no. 6, pp. 1013-1026, 2020, doi: 10.1038/s41433-019-0608-7.

[3] T. A. Bley, O. Wieben, M. Uhl, J. Thiel, D. Schmidt, and M. Langer, "High-resolution MRI in giant cell arteritis: Imaging of the wall of the superficial temporal artery," *Am. J. Roentgenol.*, vol. 184, no. 1, pp. 283-287, 2005, doi: 10.2214/ajr.184.1.01840283.

[4] F. Muratore *et al.*, "Large-vessel giant cell arteritis: A cohort study," *Rheumatol. (United Kingdom)*, vol. 54, no. 3, pp. 463-470, 2015, doi: 10.1093/rheumatology/keu329.

[5] A. Soriano, F. Muratore, N. Pipitone, L. Boiardi, L. Cimino, and C. Salvarani, "Visual loss and other cranial ischaemic complications in giant cell arteritis," *Nat. Rev. Rheumatol.*, vol. 13, no. 8, p. 476, 2017.

[6] B. Hellmich *et al.*, "2018 Update of the EULAR recommendations for the management of large vessel vasculitis," *Ann. Rheum. Dis.*, vol. 79, no. 1, pp. 19-130, 2020, doi: 10.1136/annrheumdis-2019-215672.

[7] P. W. Holm, M. Sandovici, R. H. Slart, A. W. Glaudemans, A. Rutgers, and E. Brouwer, "Vessel involvement in giant cell arteritis: an imaging approach.," *J. Cardiovasc. Surg. (Torino).*, vol. 57, no. 2, pp. 127-136, 2016.

[8] B. T. Christoph, S. Gregor, A. Markus, S. Daniel, R. Christof, and D. Thomas, "The clinical benefit of imaging in the diagnosis and treatment of giant cell arteritis," *Swiss Med. Wkly.*, vol. 148, no. 33-34, 2018, doi: 10.4414/smw.2018.14661.

[9] J. Rovenský and M. Bernadič, *Polymyalgia rheumatica and giant cell arteritis*, vol. 68, no. 4. 2019.

[10] P. W. Holm, M. Sandovici, R. H. J. A. Slart, A. W. J. M. Glaudemans, A. Rutgers, and E. Brouwer, "Vessel involvement in giant cell arteritis: An imaging approach," *J. Cardiovasc. Surg. (Torino).*, vol. 57, no. 2, pp. 127-136, 2016.

[11] Q. Zou and X. Zhou, "TI TI," 2019.

[12] X. Yang *et al.*, "Ultrasound common carotid artery segmentation based on active shape model," *Comput. Math. Methods Med.*, vol. 2013, no. Figure 1, pp. 1-12, 2013, doi: 10.1155/2013/345968.

[13] W. A. Schmidt, "Ultrasound in the diagnosis and management of giant cell arteritis," *Rheumatol. (United Kingdom)*, vol. 57, no. October 2017, pp. ii22–ii31, 2018, doi: 10.1093/rheumatology/kex461.

[14] Q. Zou, S. Ma, and X. Zhou, "Ultrasound versus temporal artery biopsy in patients with Giant cell arteritis: A prospective cohort study," *BMC Med. Imaging*, vol. 19, no. 1, pp. 1-12, 2019, doi: 10.1186/s12880-019-0344-2.

[15] R. Luqmani *et al.*, "The role of ultrasound compared to biopsy of temporal arteries in the diagnosis and treatment of giant cell arteritis (TABUL): A diagnostic accuracy and cost-effectiveness study," *Health Technol. Assess. (Rockv).*, vol. 20, no. 90, pp. 1-270, 2016, doi: 10.3310/hta20900.

[16] A. Khan and B. Dasgupta, "Imaging in Giant Cell Arteritis," *Curr. Rheumatol.*

Rep., vol. 17, no. 8, 2015, doi: 10.1007/s11926-015-0527-y.

[17] C. Duftner, C. Dejaco, A. Sepriano, L. Falzon, W. A. Schmidt, and S. Ramiro, "Imaging in diagnosis, outcome prediction and monitoring of large vessel vasculitis: A systematic literature review and meta-Analysis informing the EULAR recommendations," *RMD Open*, vol. 4, no. 1, 2018, doi: 10.1136/rmdopen-2017-000612.

[18] P. E. Berthod *et al.*, "CT analysis of the aorta in giant-cell arteritis: a case-control study," *Eur. Radiol.*, vol. 28, no. 9, pp. 3676-3684, 2018, doi: 10.1007/s00330-018-5311-8.

[19] A. Emamifar *et al.*, "The Utility of 18F-FDG PET/CT in Patients With Clinical Suspicion of Polymyalgia Rheumatica and Giant Cell Arteritis: A Prospective, Observational, and Cross-sectional Study," *ACR Open Rheumatol.*, vol. 2, no. 8, pp. 478-490, 2020, doi: 10.1002/acr2.11163.

[20] C. Dejaco *et al.*, "EULAR recommendations for the use of imaging in large vessel vasculitis in clinical practice," *Ann. Rheum. Dis.*, vol. 77, no. 5, pp. 636-643, 2018, doi: 10.1136/annrheumdis-2017-212649.

[21] K. K. Kumar, K. Chaduvula, and B. R. Markapudi, "A Detailed Survey On Feature Extraction Techniques In Image Processing For Medical Image Analysis," *Eur. J. Mol. Clin. Med.*, vol. 7, no. 10, pp. 2275-2284, 2021.

[22] S. V. M. Sagheer and S. N. George, "A review on medical image denoising algorithms," *Biomed. Signal Process. Control*, vol. 61, p. 102036, 2020.

[23] Y. Tian, Y. Pan, F. Duan, S. Zhao, Q. Wang, and W. Wang, "Automated segmentation of coronary arteries based on statistical region growing and heuristic decision method," *Biomed Res.*

Int., vol. 2016, 2016, doi: 10.1155/2016/3530251.

[24] L. A. Groves, B. VanBerlo, N. Veinberg, A. Alboog, T. M. Peters, and E. C. S. Chen, "Automatic segmentation of the carotid artery and internal jugular vein from 2D ultrasound images for 3D vascular reconstruction," *Int. J. Comput. Assist. Radiol. Surg.*, vol. 15, no. 11, pp. 1835-1846, 2020.

[25] A. Fedorov *et al.*, "3D Slicer as an image computing platform for the Quantitative Imaging Network," *Magn. Reson. Imaging*, vol. 30, no. 9, pp. 1323-1341, 2012.

[26] I. Wolf *et al.*, "The Medical Imaging Interaction Toolkit (MITK)–a toolkit facilitating the creation of interactive software by extending VTK and ITK," in *Proc. of SPIE Vol*, 2004, vol. 5367, p. 17.

[27] W. A. Schmidt, "Role of ultrasound in the understanding and management of vasculitis," *Ther. Adv. Musculoskelet. Dis.*, vol. 6, no. 2, pp. 39-47, 2014, doi: 10.1177/1759720x13512256.

[28] T. A. Bley, J. Geiger, O. Wieben, and M. Markl, "MRI of Giant Cell (Temporal) Arteritis, GCA," *MAGNETOM Flash*, 2011.

Chapter 5

Giant Cell Arteritis: From Neurologist's Perspective

Ravish Rajiv Keni, M. Sowmya and Sreekanta Swamy

Abstract

Giant cell arteritis (GCA) is a granulomatous vasculitis affecting large- and medium-sized arteries in the elderly and potentially causes visual loss. In an elderly patient presenting with acute pain in the distribution of the external carotid artery (e.g., headache, scalp tenderness); polymyalgia rhematica; or acute/transient visual loss or diplopia; a possibility of GCA should be considered in one of the differential diagnosis. Urgent laboratory evaluation (e.g., ESR, CRP, platelet count), followed immediately by empiric high-dose corticosteroid therapy is warranted in patients suspected of having GCA. Although ultrasound techniques are sensitive for the diagnosis of GCA, TAB remains the best confirmatory test. Patients with GCA often require long durations of steroid therapy and steroid-related complications are common. Multidisciplinary care and the use of steroid-sparing regimens are warranted in case of relapse.

Keywords: Giant cell arteritis, Pathogenesis, Advances, Management

1. Introduction

Giant cell arteritis (GCA) is a granulomatous vasculitis affecting medium to large sized arteries, it most commonly involves the aorta, branches of the ophthalmic artery, and extracranial branches of the carotid arteries [1–5]. From a clinical perspective, GCA is a medical emergency because if undiagnosed and treated early, ischemic complications may cause permanent vision loss in up to 15–25% of cases [6]. Early diagnosis and initiation of treatment is essential to improve visual and systemic prognosis in patients with GCA [1, 7, 8]. The complications of GCA result from ischemic injury, systemic inflammation, and aneurysm formation and rupture. Early initiation of corticosteroids in patients with suspected GCA has been found to significantly reduce the risk of permanent visual loss in various studies [6–8]. In this review we provide a brief overview regarding the pathogenesis, clinical features, investigations and management of GCA from a Neurologist's perspective.

2. Pathophysiology

GCA is immune-mediated inflammatory vasculitis affecting the medium and large-size arteries. The immunological cascade is triggered by an unknown antigen that begins with the dendritic cell processing the antigen and presenting it to T cells via the major histocompatibility complex II interaction with the T cell receptors [1, 2, 6, 9]. In this inflammatory cascade, there is downstream activation and differentiation of T cells to TH1 and TH17 cells, which in turn express interferon γ, a potent macrophage activator. This macrophage activation causes further release of chemokines including but not limited to IL-6 and tumor necrosis factor (TNF) alpha. A large number of inflammatory cells are recruited with production of reactive oxygen species (ROS) and matrix metalloproteinases (MMPs), which then primarily attack the internal elastic lamina of blood vessels. This mechanism damages the vessel wall leading to abnormal vascular remodeling and ultimately occlusion of the vessel lumen [10, 11].

2.1 Risk factors

GCA generally affects elderly population, with the average age of presentation being 74–76 years, and peak incidence at 80 years [3, 5, 9]. While GCA can occur in both men and women, it is more common in women. Women have an increased risk ranging from 2.3 to 2.6 times compared to men [1, 3, 9]. Additionally, It has been found to be affecting Caucasian ethnicity more especially those of Scandinavian, Nordic, or Northern-European ancestry [1, 3, 9]. Other important independent risk factors are smoking, early menopause and low body mass index [9, 12].

2.2 Clinical symptoms and examination findings

The symptoms of GCA include both systemic and ocular. New-onset headache is the most common systemic symptom and the systemic symptoms often precede the ocular manifestations. Fifty percent of patients with GCA have systemic symptoms and these include myalgias, headaches, scalp and temporal artery tenderness, jaw and rarely arm claudication, and constitutional symptoms (e.g., fever, anorexia, and weight loss) [1, 5]. Polymyalgia rheumatica (PMR) is present in approximately 50% of patients with biopsy-proven GCA [5]. The characteristic symptoms of PMR include: persistent pain for at least 1 month with episodes of aching and morning stiffness that lasts at least 30 minutes in the neck, shoulder, or pelvic girdle and an elevated ESR of at least 40 mm/h [5].

The most severe ocular manifestation of GCA is visual loss, with 50% of patients complaining of ocular involvement ranging from eye pain to amaurosis fugax. 19 Ocular involvement is more commonly seen in elderly patients compared to younger individuals, with no gender predilection [9, 13]. The ocular complaints include visual loss of varying severity, amaurosis fugax, diplopia, and eye pain [13]. Amaurosis fugax, precedes permanent vision loss in 44% of GCA patients [5]. Vision loss is usually mono-ocular to begin with and if left untreated, contralateral eye involvement commonly occurrs between 1 and 14 days after initial onset with the longest interval being 9 months [5, 13]. When treated early and adequately with corticosteroids, GCA-mediated blindness is preventable in majority of cases [9, 13].

In a case of suspected giant cell arteritis, the following clinical approach is recommended [4]:

- Palpation of the Temporal artery: Temporal artery may be tender, thickened and beaded. The pulse may be difficult to feel and patient may complain of scalp tenderness.

- The systemic examination should be directed at looking for evidence of large vessel vasculitis, that is looking for delayed or absent pulses in upper limbs, subclavian or carotid bruits, and blood pressure asymmetry in the limbs.

- Detailed ophthalmological exam is warranted – look for transient or permanent visual loss, visual field defect, relative afferent pupillary defect, anterior
  ischemic optic neuritis, central retinal artery occlusion.

2.3 Investigations

The following investigations are recommended in evaluation of suspected
giant cell arteritis complete blood count, renal function tests, liver function tests,
C-reactive Protein (CRP) and erythrocyte sedimentation rate (ESR) [1–5]. There
is often evidence of an acute-phase response on blood tests. Other investigations
recommended are Chest X-ray and urinalysis. Baseline (pre-treatment) markers of
inflammation are also useful to assess response to treatment.

There are a number of investigations that can also be carried out to help confirm
diagnosis, as outlined below.

- **Temporal artery biopsy**
  The gold standard for diagnosis of giant cell arteritis is Temporal artery biopsy
  (TAB). 10–20% of GCA can be biopsy negative, however a negative result
  does not rule out the condition [1–5]. The findings on temporal artery biopsy
  in GCA is characterized by inflammatory infiltration of the arterial wall by
  lymphocytes, macrophages and giant cells in about 50% of cases [1–5].

- **Temporal artery ultrasound (color-coded duplex sonography)**
  Color-coded duplex sonography can be utilized to examine the temporal,
  extracranial, occipital and subclavian arteries. An ultrasound study has a
  sensitivity of 85% and a specificity of more than 90% [1–4, 14]. The 'halo sign'
  where Inflammatory oedema of the vascular wall will be shown as hypoechoic
  wall thickening is characteristic.

- **Positron emission tomography**
  PET uses radioactive metabolites to visualize metabolic processes. Spatial
  resolution is limited with PET, so visualization can only be determined in the
  aorta and larger vessels. The ability to visualize the temporal arteries is limited
  with PET. The European League Against Rheumatism (EULAR) do not advise
  PET to screen the cranial vessels, however by using newer PET scanners with
  improved spatial resolution the temporal arteries may be better visualized in
  the future [15, 16].

- **High-resolution magnetic resonance imaging**
  For imaging of temporal arteries MRI is the imaging modality of choice recommended by the EULAR [16]. Detailed imaging of the walls and lumen of the
  temporal artery is possible by doing a High-resolution MRI (fat suppression,
  T1 weighted) allows. A concurrent MR angiography allows imaging of large
  vessels such as aorta and sub-clavian artery.

3. Diagnosis of GCA

Diagnosis of GCA is based on clinical and laboratory tests and application of the
revised ACR criteria (**Table 1**) [17]. It has been suggested that in the presence of 3
points or more out of 11, with at least 1 point belonging to Domain 1, the diagnosis
of GCA can be established.

SCORE	
N/A	Age at onset ≥50 years old
	Absence of exclusion criteria[b]
DOMAIN I	
1	New onset localized headache[c]
1	Sudden onset of visual disturbances[c]
2	Polymyalgia Rheumatica
1	Jaw Claudication[c]
2	Abnormal temporal artery[d] up to 2 points
DOMAIN II	
1	Unexplained fever and/or anemia 1 point
1	ESR ≥50 mm/hour[e] 1p
2	Compatible pathology[f] up to 2 points

[a]*In the presence of 3 points or more out of 11 with at least one point belonging to domain I along with all entry criteria, the diagnosis of Giant cell arteritis can be established.*
[b]*Exclusion criteria are including: ENT and eye inflammation, kidney, skin and peripheral nervous system involvement, lung infiltration, lymphadenopathies, stiff neck and digital gangrene or ulceration.*
[c]*No other aetiologies can better explain any one of the criteria.*
[d]*-Enlarged and/or pulseless temporal artery: 1 point/tender temporal artery: 1 point.*
[e]*It must be ignored in the presence of PMR.*
[f]*Vascular and/or perivascular fibrinoid necrosis along with leucocyte infiltration: 1 point and granuloma: 1 point.*

Table 1.
Revised ACR criteria (rACR) for diagnosis of GCA[a] [17].

4. Treatment

4.1 Corticosteroids

Initiation of prompt corticosteroid treatment is recommended [1–5]. In cases where there is a clinical suspicion of giant cell arteritis, corticosteroid treatment should be initiated immediately and not delayed awaiting results of blood tests or temporal artery biopsy.

In cases of complicated giant cell arteritis, that is when there is evolving visual loss or amaurosis fugax: Intravenous methylprednisolone in a dosage of 500 mg–1 g IV for three days followed by corticosteroid dose is advised.

A corticosteroid tapering regimen is suggested below [18]:

- Start with prednisolone 40–60 mg daily continue for at least three to four weeks until clinical symptoms and laboratory abnormalities begin to resolve

- Subsequently reduce the dose by 10 mg every two weeks to 20 mg daily, followed by further reduction of dose by 2.5 mg every two to four weeks to 10 mg daily

- Subsequently it is recommended to reduce the dose by 1 mg every one to two months, provided the condition does not relapse again.

Corticosteroids can generally be reduced when the clinical features of active disease are absent and when the laboratory markers for acute inflammation such as ESR, C-reactive protein are normalized.

4.2 Aspirin

The usage of Aspirin is controversial; albeit it remains in the recommendations [18], when not contraindicated. Aspirin has been found to be protective against cerebrovascular and cardiovascular events in previous studies [19]. Apart from its antiplatelet effects and Aspirin also has disease-modifying effects through suppression of interferon (IFN) gamma [18, 19].

4.3 Management of relapse

All patients with suspected relapse should be referred to, or have their treatment discussed with, a specialist [1–5, 18, 19]. In case of relapse, a rise in inflammatory markers (ESR/CRP) is usually seen, however these markers can remain normal in some cases. In case of recurrence of headache, the patient should revert to the previous higher corticosteroid dosage. In case of jaw claudication, a prednisolone dosage of 60 mg daily is recommended. Ocular symptoms need prednisolone 60 mg daily orally or intravenous pulse methylprednisolone 1 g and immediate opthalmology consultation.

4.4 Management of Recurrent relapse

Despite an initial good response to therapy, about 30–50% of patients will suffer a relapse, within the next two years [1–5, 18–20]. The use of secondary agents such as methotrexate (or others such as azathioprine in patients, who are intolerant to methotrexate) should be considered in patients with recurrent relapse or failure. Various clinical trials have shown that Methotrexate (7.5–15 mg once a week) reduces the relapse rate and overall duration of exposure to corticosteroids [20].

4.5 Tocilizumab

Tocilizumab is an interleukin-6 (IL-6)-receptor inhibitor. The Giant Cell Arteritis Actemra (GiACTA) trial demonstrated increased rates of sustained remission using a combination of tocilizumab plus corticosteroids compared with those treated with corticosteroids alone [21]. Furthermore, steroid-induced adverse effects were reduced with the usage of tocilizumab for treatment.

Tocilizumab is recommended by NICE as an option for treating GCA in adults, in case they have relapsing, or refractory disease and they have not already taken tocilizumab; it is stopped after one year of uninterrupted treatment at most [20].

Tocilizumab is a potent suppressor of IL-6, which is important producer of CRP. Therefore, patients on tocilizumab may not produce a biochemical inflammatory response in the setting of infection/inflammation. Caution should be taken while taking Tocilizumab, particularly in patients with a history of diverticulitis, as it carries a risk for gastrointestinal perforation [22].

5. Conclusion

In an elderly patient presenting with acute pain in the distribution of the external carotid artery (e.g., headache, scalp tenderness); PMR; or acute/transient visual loss or diplopia; a possibility of GCA should be considered in one of the differential diagnosis. Urgent laboratory evaluation (e.g., ESR, CRP, platelet count), followed immediately by empiric high-dose corticosteroid therapy is warranted in patients suspected of having GCA. Although ultrasound techniques are sensitive for the diagnosis of GCA, TAB remains the best confirmatory test. Patients with GCA often require long durations of steroid therapy and steroid-related complications are common. Multidisciplinary care and the use of steroid-sparing regimens is warranted in case of relapse.

Disclosure

The authors report no conflicts of interest in this work.

Author details

Ravish Rajiv Keni*, M. Sowmya and Sreekanta Swamy
Department of Neurology, Aster RV Hospital, Bengaluru, India

*Address all correspondence to: ravish81284@gmail.com

IntechOpen

References

[1] Hayreh SS, Zimmerman B. Management of giant cell arteritis. Ophthalmologica. 2003; 217(4):239-259.

[2] Rahman W, Rahman FZ, Cell G. Giant cell (temporal) arteritis: an overview and update. Surv Ophthalmol. 2005;50(5):415-428.

[3] Hoffman GS, Arteritis GC. Giant cell arteritis. Ann Intern Med. 2016;165(9):ITC65.

[4] El-Dairi MA, Chang L, Proia AD, Cummings TJ, Stinnett SS, Bhatti MT. Diagnostic algorithm for patients with suspected giant cell arteritis. J Neuroophthalmol. 2015;35(3):246-253.

[5] Salvarani C, Cantini F, Boiardi L, Hunder GG. Polymyalgia rheumatica and giant-cell arteritis. N Engl J Med. 2002;347(4):261-271.

[6] Patil P, Williams M, Maw WW, et al. Fast track pathway reduces sight loss in giant cell arteritis: results of a longitudinal observational cohort study. Clin Exp Rheumatol. 2015;33(2 Suppl 89):S-103-6.

[7] Hocevar A, Rotar Z, Jese R, et al. Do early diagnosis and glucocorticoid treatment decrease the risk of permanent visual loss and early relapses in giant cell arteritis: a prospective longitudinal study. Medicine. 2016;95(14):e3210.

[8] Diamantopoulos AP, Haugeberg G, Lindland A, Myklebust G. The fast-track ultrasound clinic for early diagnosis of giant cell arteritis significantly reduces permanent visual impairment: towards a more effective strategy to improve clinical outcome in giant cell arteritis? Rheumatology. 2016;55(1):66-70.

[9] Baig IF, Pascoe AR, Kini A, Lee AG. Giant cell arteritis: early diagnosis is key. Eye Brain. 2019;11:1-12.

[10] Cid MC. 3. Pathogenesis of giant cell arteritis. Rheumatology. 2014;53 (suppl 2):i2–i3. https://doi.org/.

[11] Hernández-Rodríguez J, Segarra M, Vilardell C, et al. Tissue production of pro-inflammatory cytokines (IL-1beta, TNFalpha and IL-6) correlates with the intensity of the systemic inflammatory response and with corticosteroid requirements in giant-cell arteritis. Rheumatology. 2004;43(3):294-301.

[12] Larsson K, Mellström D, Nordborg E, Nordborg C, Odén A, Nordborg E. Early menopause, low body mass index, and smoking are independent risk factors for developing giant cell arteritis. Ann Rheum Dis. 2006;65(4):529-532.

[13] Hayreh SS, Podhajsky PA, Zimmerman B. Ocular manifestations of giant cell arteritis. Am J Ophthalmol. 1998;125(4):509-520.

[14] Ness T, Bley TA, Schmidt WA, Lamprecht P. The diagnosis and treatment of giant cell arteritis. Dtsch Arztebl Int. 2013 May;110(21):376-385; quiz 386.

[15] Blockmans D. The use of (18F) fluoro-deoxyglucose positron emission tomography in the assessment of large vessel vasculitis. Clin Exp Rheumatol 2009;21:15-22.

[16] Dejaco C, Ramiro S, Duftner C, et al. EULAR recommendations for the use of imaging in large vessel vasculitis in clinical practice. Ann Rheum Dis. 2018;77(5):636-643.

[17] I Salehi-Abari. 2016 ACR revised criteria for early diagnosis of giant cell (temporal) arteritis. Autoimmune Dis Ther Approaches Open Access 2016;3:1-4.

[18] Dasgupta B, Borg FA, Hassan N, et al. BSR and BHPR guidelines for

the management of giant cell arteritis. Rheumatology (Oxford). 2010;49(8): 1594-1597.

[19] Nesher G, Berkun Y, Mates M, Baras M, Rubinow A, Sonnenblick M. Low-dose aspirin and prevention of cranial ischemic complications in giant cell arteritis. Arthritis Rheum. 2004 Apr;50(4):1332-1337.

[20] Mahr AD, Jover JA, Spiera RF, et al. Adjunctive methotrexate for treatment of giant cell arteritis: an individual patient data meta-analysis. Arthritis Rheum. 2007 Aug;56(8):2789-2797.

[21] Stone JH, Tuckwell K, Dimonaco S, et al. Trial of tocilizumab in giant-cell arteritis. N Engl J Med Overseas Ed. 2017;377(4):317-328.

[22] Gout T, Ostör AJ, Nisar MK. Lower gastrointestinal perforation in rheumatoid arthritis patients treated with conventional DMARDs or tocilizumab: a systematic literature review. Clin Rheumatol. 2011; 30(11):1471-1474.

Chapter 6

Clinical Manifestations of Giant Cell Arteritis

Ryan Costa Silva, Inês Silva, Joana Rodrigues Santos,
Tania Vassalo, Joana Rosa Martins and Ligia Peixoto

Abstract

Giant cell arteritis (GCA), also known as temporal arteritis or Horton disease, is categorized as a large- and medium-sized vessels vasculitis. Systemic symptoms are common in GCA and although vascular involvement may be widespread, the cranial branches of the aortic arch are responsible for the hallmark symptoms of GCA: headache, jaw claudication and ocular symptoms, particularly visual loss. The large vessel (LV)-GCA phenotype may differ or overlap from cranial arteritis. Clinical consequences of LV-GCA comprise aneurysms and dissections of the aorta, as well as stenosis, occlusion and ectasia of large arteries. Symptoms of polymyalgia rheumatica occurring in a patient with GCA include characteristic proximal polyarthralgias and myalgias, sometimes accompanied by remitting seronegative symmetrical synovitis with pitting edema (RS3PE), Less common manifestations reported include central nervous system involvement, audiovestibular and upper respiratory symptoms, pericarditis, mesenteric ischemia and female genital tract involvement.

Keywords: systemic symptoms, cranial arteritis, headaches, visual disturbance, vision loss, polymyalgia rheumatica, RS3PE, large vessel phenotype

1. Introduction

Giant cell arteritis (GCA), also known as temporal arteritis or Horton disease, is a systemic inflammatory large-vessel vasculitis that usually affects the aorta and its major branches [1].

The pathophysiology of GCA is complex and not fully understood. Histopathology studies reveal inflammation of the artery wall with predominance of CD4+ T lymphocytes and macrophages, which frequently undergo granulomatous organization with formation of giant cells. Immunopathology and molecular studies performed with temporal artery biopsies have led to the current pathogenic model [2].

GCA is primarily an immune-mediated disease due to a maladaptive response to endothelial injury, occurring in susceptible individuals and triggered by factors that have not been identified with certainty. Several microbe and viral sequences, including varicella-zoster virus, have been detected in temporal artery lesions, but no convincing causal relationship has been demonstrated [3].

The initial inflammatory response involves the activation of dendritic cells, present in the adventitia of normal arteries, through pathogen- or damage-sensing receptors, such as toll-like receptors, producing chemokines able to attract and retain dendritic cells as well as lymphocytes and macrophages. Once activated, dendritic cells are enabled to process and present antigens and strongly express major histocompatability complex (MHC) class II and costimulatory molecules (CD83 and CD86) required for T-cell recruitment [4].

Once activated, both T helper (Th)1 and Th17 differentiation pathways contribute to the development of vascular inflammation. Interleukin (IL)-12 and IL-18 produced by dendritic cells stimulate Th1 differentiation and production of interferon (IFN)-gamma which is noticeably expressed in GCA-involved arteries. IFN-gamma causes endothelial cells and vascular smooth muscle to recruit more Th1 cells, CD8+ T cells, and monocytes which differentiate into macrophages and the characteristic giant cells that produce growth factors, interleukins and proteolytic enzymes playing a distinctive role granuloma formation that progressively narrow and obstruct the vessel wall [5].

Moreover, IL-1-beta, IL-6, and IL-21 promote Th17 differentiation, which is maintained by IL-23 and results in IL-17A expression. IL-17A, profusely expressed in GCA lesions, is a proinflammatory cytokine having pleiotropic effects on a variety of cells, namely macrophages, fibroblasts, endothelial cells and vascular smooth muscle cells [6].

Systemic manifestations are related the inflammatory process and cytokine amplification. Inflammation-induced vascular remodeling leads to concentric intimal hyperplasia occurring as a repair mechanism in response to injury of the blood vessel wall. End-organ involvement results from mural hyperplasia which can narrow the arterial lumen, resulting in distal ischemia and ischemic complications of the disease [7].

2. Clinical manifestations of giant cell arteritis

Clinical presentation of GCA tends to be subacute, but may occur over the course of a few days. Although symptoms of GCA are nonspecific, some key findings may strongly suggest this diagnosis. Systemic symptoms are common in GCA and vascular involvement can be widespread, causing stenosis and aneurysm of affected vessels. It is the targeting of the tiny muscular arteries from cranial branches of the aortic arch, however, that gives rise to many of the most characteristic symptoms of GCA. External carotid branch involvement accounts for the high frequency of cranial symptoms [8].

2.1 Constitutional symptoms

Systemic symptoms associated with GCA are frequent and include fever, fatigue, anorexia and weight loss. These symptoms may occur for a few days and may prolong to several weeks. Fever is usually low grade and occurs in up to one-half of patients. It has been stated as well that 1 out of 6 fevers of unknown origin in older adults was due to GCA [9]. About 10% of patients with GCA present with constitutional symptoms and laboratory evidence of inflammation as the only clues to the diagnosis [10]. Thus, in an older adult with fever or constitutional symptoms not explained by an initial evaluation for infection or malignancy, a diagnosis of GCA warrants consideration [11].

2.2 Headache

Headache is a common presentation of GCA, being the initial symptom in 33% of cases and present in about 80% of patients [12]. Importantly, the headache is either new, in a patient without previous history of headaches, or of a new type in a patient with chronic headache.

While the headache has no pathognomonic features, headaches due to GCA are typically throbbing and continuous, located over the temples, but can also be frontal, occipital, unilateral or generalized. Descriptions of the pain range from a dull or burning sensation to focal tenderness on direct palpation. Patients may note scalp tenderness with hair combing or when wearing a hat. The headache can progressively worsen, wax and wane, or sometimes recede before treatment is started [13].

2.3 Jaw claudication

Jaw claudication results from ischemia of the maxillary artery supplying the masseter muscles and is highly predictive of temporal arteritis. Nearly 50% of patients experience jaw claudication, a symptom consisting of mandibular pain, discomfort or fatigue triggered by mastication or prolonged speaking and relieved by stopping [14]. An analysis of the diagnostic value of temporal artery biopsies, which correlated positive biopsies with clinical symptoms, revealed jaw claudication as the symptom most highly associated with a positive biopsy [15].

In some cases, patients note a trismus-like symptom, with either perceived or actual limitation of temporomandibular joint excursion. Claudication symptoms occasionally affect the tongue, with repeated swallowing and tongue infarction being almost pathognomonic for GCA [16, 17].

2.4 Ocular involvement

The reported incidence of visual symptoms in GCA ranges widely [18]. These include permanent visual loss, transient monocular (and, rarely, binocular) vision impairment, consisting of unilateral visual blurring, vision loss or diplopia. Patients refer an abrupt partial field defect or temporary curtain effect in the field of vision of one eye [19]. It can be useful in the course of evaluating the possible significance of a reported visual disturbance to inquire if the patient tried to cover each eye since explicit monocular visual loss would heighten concern for GCA. Transient visual loss can be a harbinger of permanent visual loss, especially if treatment is not started promptly and thus mandates urgent attention in a patient with suspected GCA.

The most feared complication of GCA is permanent loss of vision, frequently sudden and painless, may be partial or complete, and may be unilateral or bilateral. Permanent loss of vision in GCA results from arteritic anterior ischemic optic neuropathy, central or branch retinal artery occlusion, posterior ischemic optic neuropathy, or, rarely, cerebral ischemia [20]. Even in the current era effective therapy, the incidence of permanent loss of vision ranged from 15 to 20% of patients [20]. Though permanent visual loss may be preceded by single or multiple episodes of transient visual loss, it can also occur with devastating swiftness. When untreated, contralateral eye involvement commonly occurs between the first two weeks after initial onset [21]. With adequate glucocorticoid treatment, if there is no further visual deterioration within the first week, existing vision in affected eye and the vision in the unaffected eye will remain intact, virtually stopping the subsequent risk of sight loss [22].

Extraocular motility disorders occur in approximately 5% of atients and include diplopia which has a high specificity when accompanied by other symptoms suggestive of GCA [23]. Diplopia, which is usually transient, can result from ischemia of any portion of the oculomotor system, including the brainstem, oculomotor nerves, and the extraocular muscles themselves [24].

Although rare, GCA can manifest with Charles Bonnet syndrome, a phenomenon of visual hallucinations in psychologically normal individuals who have visual loss due to lesions in either peripheral or central visual pathways [25].

2.5 Musculoskeletal involvement

GCA is closely linked to polymyalgia rheumatica (PMR) and this well-known association has therapeutic and prognostic consequences. About 40 to 60% of GCA patients have manifestations of PMR, an inflammatory rheumatic condition clinically characterized by symmetrical proximal polyarthralgia and myalgia, with aching and stiffness on shoulders, hip girdle, neck, torso and an unfamiliar sense of fatigue [26].

Less commonly, distal findings can occur, involving synovitis of peripheral joints, especially at the wrists and metacarpophalangeal joints, with distal extremity swelling and pitting edema, known as remitting seronegative symmetrical synovitis with pitting edema (RS3PE) syndrome, puffy edematous hand syndrome or distal extremity swelling with pitting edema [27]. In this syndrome symptoms can appear abruptly, with significant swelling, usually pitting, extending over the dorsal side of the wrists and metacarpophalangeal joints producing a "boxing glove" appearance, and with limited range of motion of the hands and wrists. The term seronegative refers to the absence of antibodies namely rheumatoid factor (RF) and cyclic citrullinated peptide (anti-CCP) for differential diagnosis with rheumatoid arthritis. Imaging with ultrasonography and MRI reveal tenosynovitis of the extensor tendon of the forearms and hands, with less flexor tenosynovitis and synovitis of the metacarpophalangeal and proximal interphalangeal joints [28]. A paraneoplastic association with solid tumors and hematologic disorders has been reported, but in clinical practice such an occurrence is rare [29].

2.6 Large vessel involvement

Involvement of the extracranial branches of the carotid artery is the source of the classic cranial symptoms of GCA. However, besides the carotid arteries, GCA often involves the aorta and its major branches which is designated large vessel (LV) -GCA. The clinical consequences of LV-GCA include aneurysms and dissections of the aorta, particularly the thoracic aorta, as well as stenosis, occlusion, and ectasia of large arteries. This subset of patients with predominantly upper extremity arterial vasculitis, may have variable clinical presentations and diagnostic delay [30].

While symptomatic LV involvement is uncommon, a key point is that subclinical LV-GCA involvement is present in a significant number of patients and can underlie a systemic presentation of GCA without having necessarily cranial symptomatology. Different publications using imaging modalities such as fluorodeoxyglucose positron emission tomography (FDG-PET), computed tomographic (CT) angiography and color-coded duplex ultrasonography have consistently highlighted the involvement of subclavian, axillary, brachial arteries or the thoracic aorta in more than 30% of patients with confirmed GCA diagnosis [31, 32].

Although the disease pattern of LV-GCA differs from cranial GCA, clinical features overlap. Systematic screening of patients with the cranial phenotype can demonstrate large artery involvement. On the other hand, temporal artery biopsies are positive in only approximately one-half of patients with LV GCA, underlining the essential role of imaging for the diagnosis of this phenotype.

In contrast with the cranial phenotype, LV-GCA patients were younger at disease onset (66 vs. 72 years), had longer duration of symptoms prior to the diagnosis (median 3.5 months vs. 2.2 months), fewer cranial symptoms (41% vs. 83%) and were more likely to have arm claudication at presentation (51% vs. 0%) [33].

Aortic aneurysms have been recognized in 10% of cases [34]. The thoracic aorta is more frequently affected than the abdominal aorta, and within the thoracic aorta the descending segment is the main site. It is important to note that in these cases, there is often little or no clinical or laboratory evidence of systemic activity of GCA. When compared with the general population, patients with GCA have a twofold increased risk of aortic aneurysm and this should be considered within the range of other risk factors such as male gender, age or smoking [35]. Histopathologic examination of specimens from surgery or autopsy show fibrosis and different degrees of active aortitis, including giant cells. These findings suggest two mechanisms of disease: chronic recrudescent aortitis causing elastin and collagen disruption, or mechanical stress on an aortic wall weakened in the early active phase of the disease. Aortic dissection or rupture is a rare major complication of aortitis and was identified in 5% of patients with LV-GCA with aortic aneurysm [36]. Involvement of the ascending aorta can lead to aortic rupture, and coronary arteritis may result in myocardial infarction.

GCA can also affect the subclavian arteries distal to the take-off of the vertebral arteries and extend through the axillary arteries to the proximal brachial arteries. On physical examination, arterial bruits, diminished or absent blood pressures and arm claudication can be identified. Cold intolerance of the involved extremity is common, but explicit digital ulcerations and gangrene are rare because of adequate collateral arterial supply. The vessel wall is circumferentially affected, in contrast to the eccentric appearance of atherosclerosis. The descending aorta and mesenteric, renal, iliac, and femoral arteries can less commonly be affected, with attendant complications of intestinal infarction, renal infarction, crural infarction and ischemic mononeuropathies [37]. Clinically evident lower-extremity arterial involvement can occur but is also uncommon [38].

2.7 Central nervous system involvement

Stroke is a rare but important complication of GCA and is typically due to stenosis of carotid and the vertebral or basilar arteries. Even with aggressive steroid and immunosuppressive therapy it is associated with high morbidity and mortality. In descriptive cohorts, the frequency of stroke within the first four weeks of the diagnosis of GCA, and thus construed as potentially disease-related, has ranged from 1.5 to 7.5% [39].

Though strokes due to GCA can occur in the distribution of both the internal carotid and vertebrobasilar arteries, they are noticeably more frequent in the latter location. More than one-half of strokes attributable to GCA occur in the vertebrobasilar system This figure contrasts with population-based studies of transient ischemic attacks and stroke overall, which occur five times more often in the territory of the internal carotid arteries compared with the vertebrobasilar arteries [40]. Arteritic involvement of the vertebral arteries can result in vertigo, ataxia, dysarthria, homonymous hemianopsia, or bilateral cortical blindness. Bilateral vertebral artery involvement, which causes rapidly progressive brainstem or cerebellar neurologic deficits with high mortality, is highly suggestive of GCA.

Peripheral neuropathy, myelopathy, higher cortical dysfunction or dementia, and pachymeningitis are uncommon complications of GCA.

2.8 Respiratory tract symptoms

Patients with GCA can present upper respiratory tract symptoms, in particular a non-productive cough. The cause of cough is unknown, but may result from vasculitis in the area of cough receptors, which are located throughout the respiratory tree, or vasculitis of the ascending pharyngeal artery, a branch of the external carotid artery. Vasculitis of the bronchial arteries has been observed in the post-mortem examination of a patient with disseminated GCA. Furthermore, involvement of the lungs in GCA has also been reported as cases of interstitial lung disease (ILD) as an uncommon clinical manifestation of GCA [41].

2.9 Cardiac involvement

Patients with GCA are at increased risk for cardiovascular events, but cardiac involvement is rare. Myocardial infarction is an example of serious complication that may arise. Cases of GCA patients developing myocarditis and myopericarditis are uncommon but have been reported [42].

2.10 Head and neck involvement

Branches of the external carotid artery may often be affected in GCA, namely the superficial temporal artery. Jaw claudication results from arteritic involvement of the muscles of mastication (masseter, temporalis, and medial and lateral ptery-goid muscles), all of which are supplied by the branches of the external carotid artery. Involvement of other branches of the external carotid artery accounts for many of the other extracranial symptoms that can accompany the presentation of GCA, including: maxillary and dental pain, facial swelling, throat pain, tongue pain and macroglossia [43].

2.11 Atypical features

GCA of the female genital tract was first reported by Ritawa in 1951 [44]. Female genital tract involvement (ovary, fallopian tubes, or uterus) was identified by chance on histopathologic inspection of surgical specimens surgically removed for gynecological reasons unrelated to GCA.

Vasculitis of the breast does occur and should require exclusion of systemic involvement. When constitutional symptoms, especially arthralgia and myalgia, are present and acute phase reactants are elevated, a work-up for systemic disease is especially warranted. Histologic characteristics included vessel size and type of inflammatory infiltrates including foamy macrophages and giant cells [45]. These features did not correlate with disease extent, plus constitutional and musculoskeletal manifestations were usually absent. Patients generally did not require systemic therapy and may be cured by resection alone.

3. Conclusion

GCA should always be considered in the differential diagnosis of a new-onset headache in patients 50 years of age or older with an elevated erythrocyte sedimentation rate. Temporal artery biopsy remains the criterion standard for diagnosis of this granulomatous vasculitis but increasing evidence supports the use of imaging studies such as ultrasonography as a less invasive from of diagnosis.

The onset of symptoms in GCA tends to be subacute, but abrupt presentations occur in some patients. Although systemic manifestations are characteristic of GCA and although vascular involvement can be widespread, clinical manifestations of the disease most frequently result from involvement of the cranial branches of arteries originating from the aortic arch. When taking the patient's history, the clinician must ask about the following types of symptoms: systemic symptoms, such as fever, fatigue, and weight loss; headache; jaw claudication, which is the symptom most highly predictive of a positive temporal artery for the diagnosis of GCA; visual symptoms, particularly transient monocular visual loss and diplopia. The most threatening complication of GCA, visual loss, is a potential result of the cranial phenotype arteritis.

A close relationship exists between GCA and PMR but the precise nature of this association is poorly understood. Several authors have suggested that these two entities are actually different stages of the same disease process. Symptoms of polymyalgia rheumatica occurring in a patient with GCA include characteristic proximal polyarthralgias and myalgias, sometimes accompanied by remitting seronegative symmetrical synovitis with pitting edema (RS3PE).

Most GCA patients present with clinical manifestations that are the result of vascular involvement but a variable proportion of patients may present without obvious vascular manifestations. Imaging may be particularly helpful in the diagnosis of GCA of large arteries in patients with atypical or occult GCA disease. Subclinical involvement of the aorta and large arteries is frequent, a clinical consequence of which can be aortic aneurysm which rarely can be complicated with dissection or rupture. Measurement of the blood pressures in both arms and careful assessment of the arterial tree by palpation and auscultation should be performed in all patients with suspected GCA. When compared with cranial disease, LV-GCA patients have higher relapse rate, greater corticosteroid requirements and increased prevalence of aortic aneurysm. It should be noted that both the 1990 and the revised 2016 American College of Rheumatology criteria may fail to recognize the LV-GCA phenotype, since a portion of LV-GCA do not have cranial symptoms.

The major risk factor for developing giant cell arteritis is aging. The disease almost never occurs before age 50 years, and its incidence rises steadily thereafter. Giant cell arteritis is a more heterogeneous condition than previously thought. Clear knowledge of all the potential clinical manifestations is essential to avoid a delayed diagnosis and associated complications. Although most of these manifestations occur prior to steroid therapy, they may also develop during the early phase of therapy or relapse with tapering of the dose of steroids. Earlier diagnosis, close monitoring and improving the treatment protocols may prevent mortality and improve morbidity in these cases.

Funding

No funding was received for the development of this paper.

Conflict of interest

The authors declare no conflict of interest.

Author details

Ryan Costa Silva*, Inês Silva, Joana Rodrigues Santos, Tania Vassalo,
Joana Rosa Martins and Ligia Peixoto
Centro Hospitalar Universitario Lisboa Norte, Hospital de Santa Maria, Lisboa,
Portugal

*Address all correspondence to: ryansilva@campus.ul.pt

IntechOpen

References

[1] Ciofalo A, Gulotta G, Iannella G, et al. Giant Cell Arteritis (GCA): pathogenesis, clinical aspects and treatment approaches. Curr Rheumatol Rev. 2019; 15(4):259-268.

[2] Terrades-Garcia N, Cid MC. Pathogenesis of giant-cell arteritis: How targeted therapies are influencing our understanding of the mechanisms involved. Rheumatology (Oxford) 2018; 57:ii51.

[3] Procop GW, Eng C, Clifford A, et al. Varicella Zoster Virus and Large Vessel Vasculitis, the Absence of an Association. Pathog Immun 2017; 2:228.

[4] Samson M, Corbera-Bellalta M, Audia S, Planas-Rigol E, Martin L, Cid MC, et al. Recent advances in our understanding of giant cell arteritis pathogenesis. Autoimmun Rev 2017;16(8):833-844.

[5] Dinkin M, Johnson E. One giant step for giant cell arteritis: updates in diagnosis and treatment. Curr Treat Options Neurol. 2021; 23(2):6.

[6] Régent A, Ly KH, Mouthon L. Physiopathology of giant cell arteritis: from inflammation to vascular remodeling. Presse Med. 2019; 48(9):919-930.

[7] Dejaco C, Brouwer E, Mason JC, et al. Giant cell arteritis and olymyalgia rheumatica: current challenges and opportunities. Nat Rev Rheumatol 2017; 13:578.

[8] Salvarani C, Cantini F, Hunder GG. Polymyalgia rheumatica and giant-cell arteritis. Lancet 2008; 372:234-245.

[9] Knockaert DC, Vanneste LJ, Bobbaers HJ. Fever of unknown origin in elderly patients. J Am Geriatr Soc 1993; 41:1187.

[10] Talarico R, Stagnaro C, Ferro F, et al. Giant cell arteritis presenting as fever of unknown origin and delay in diagnosis: analysis of two different decades. Annals of the Rheumatic Diseases 2020;79:694.

[11] Poudel P, Swe T, Wiilliams M, et al. Fever as the sole presentation of giant cell arteritis: a near miss. J Investig Med High Impact Case Rep. 2019; 7:2324709619850222.

[12] Gonzalez-Gay MA, Barros S, Lopez-Diaz MJ, et al. Giant cell arteritis: disease patterns of clinical presentation in a series of 240 patients. Medicine (Baltimore) 2005; 84:269.

[13] Mollan SP, Paemeleire K, Versijpt J, et al. European Headache Federation recommendations for neurologists managing giant cell arteritis. J Headache Pain. 2020; 21(1):28.

[14] van der Geest KSM, Sandovici M, Brouwer E, et al. Diagnostic accuracy of symptoms, physical signs, and laboratory tests for giant cell arteritis: a systematic review and meta-analysis. JAMA Intern Med. 2020; 180(10):1295-1304.

[15] Gabriel SE, O'Fallon WM, Achkar AA, et al. The use of clinical characteristics to predict the results of temporal artery biopsy among patients with suspected giant cell arteritis. J Rheumatol 1995; 22:93.

[16] Kuo CH, McCluskey P, Fraser CL. Chewing Gum Test for Jaw Claudication in Giant-Cell Arteritis. N Engl J Med. 2016 May 5. 374 (18):1794-5.

[17] Bhatti MT, Frohman L, Nesher G. MD Roundtable: Diagnosing Giant Cell Arteritis. EyeNet. 2017 June. 21(6):31-34.

[18] Ivana Vodopivec, Joseph F Rizzo. Ophthalmic manifestations of giant cell

arteritis. Rheumatology (Oxford) 2018; 57:ii63-72.

[19] Tadi P, Najem K, Margolin E. Amaurosis Fugax. StatPearls Publishing 2020.

[20] Chen JJ, Leavitt JA, Fang C, et al. Evaluating the incidence of arteritic ischemic optic neuropathy and other causes of vision loss from giant cell arteritis. Ophthalmology. 2016 Sep. 123(9):1999-2003.

[21] Baig IF, Pascoe AR, Kini A, et al. Giant cell arteritis: early diagnosis is key. Eye Brain. 2019;11:1-12.

[22] Baig IF, Pascoe AR, Kini A, et al. Giant cell arteritis: early diagnosis is key. Eye Brain. 2019;11:1-12.

[23] Smetana GW, Shmerling RH. Does this patient have temporal arteritis? JAMA 2002; 287:92.

[24] Vodopivec I, Rizzo JF. Ophthalmic manifestations of giant cell arteritis. Rheumatology (Oxford) 2018; 57:ii63.

[25] Bloch J, Morell-Dubois S, Koch E et al. Visual hallucinations and giant cell arteritis: the Charles Bonnet syndrome. Rev Med Interne. 2011 Dec; 32(12):e119-21

[26] Salvarani C, Cantini F, Hunder G. Polymyalgia rheumatica and giant-cell arteritis. Lancet. 2008; 372:234-245.

[27] Smets P, Devauchelle-Pensec V, Rouzaire PO, et al. Vascular endothelial growth factor levels and rheumatic diseases of the elderly. Arthritis Res Ther. 2016 Dec 1;18(1):283.

[28] Klauser A, Frauscher F, Halpern E, et al. Remitting seronegative symmetrical synovitis with pitting edema of the hands: ultrasound, doppler ultrasound and magnetic resonance imaging findings. Arthritis Rheum 2005; 53:226.

[29] Sibilia J, Friess S, Schaeverbeke T, et al. Remitting seronegative symmetrical synovitis with pitting edema (RS3PE): a form of paraneoplastic polyarthritis? J Rheumatol 1999; 26:115.

[30] Muratore F, Kermani TA, Crowson CS, et al. Large-vessel giant cell arteritis: a cohort study. Rheumatology (Oxford). 2015 Mar; 54(3):463-70.

[31] Blockmans D, de Ceuninck L, Vanderschueren S, et al. Repetitive 18F-fluorodeoxyglucose positron emission tomography in giant cell arteritis: a prospective study of 35 patients. Arthritis Rheum 2006; 55:131.

[32] Ghinoi A, Pipitone N, Nicolini A, et al. Large-vessel involvement in recent-onset giant cell arteritis: a case-control colour-Doppler sonography study. Rheumatology (Oxford) 2012; 51:730.

[33] Brack A, Martinez-Taboada V, Stanson A, et al. Disease pattern in cranial and large-vessel giant cell arteritis. Arthritis Rheum 1999; 42:311.

[34] Kebed DT, Bois JP, Connolly HM, et al. Spectrum of Aortic Disease in the Giant Cell Arteritis Population. Am J Cardiol 2018; 121:501.

[35] Robson JC, Kiran A, Maskell J, et al. The relative risk of aortic aneurysm in patients with giant cell arteritis compared with the general population of the UK. Ann Rheum Dis 2015; 74:129.

[36] Nuenninghoff DM, Hunder GG, Christianson TJ, et al. Incidence and predictors of large-artery complication (aortic aneurysm, aortic dissection, and/or large-artery stenosis) in patients with giant cell arteritis: a population-based study over 50 years. Arthritis Rheum 2003; 48:3522.

[37] Scola CJ, Li C, Upchurch KS. Mesenteric involvement in giant

cell arteritis. An underrecognized complication? Analysis of a case series with clinicoanatomic correlation. Medicine (Baltimore). 2008 Jan. 87(1):45-51.

[38] Kelly NP, Vaidya A, Herman M, et al. An Unusual Cause of Leg Pain. N Engl J Med 2017; 377:e29.

[39] Gonzalez MA, Rodriguez TR, Acebo I, et al. Strokes at time of disease diagnosis in a series of 287 patients with biopsy-proven giant cell arteritis. Medicine (Baltimore) 2009; 88:227.

[40] Turney TM, Garraway WM, Whisnant JP. The natural history of hemispheric and brainstem infarction in Rochester, Minnesota. Stroke 1984; 15:790.

[41] Konishi C, Nakagawa K, Nakai E, et al. Interstitial Lung Disease as an Initial Manifestation of Giant Cell Arteritis. Intern Med 2017; 56(19): 2633-2637.

[42] Bablekos GD, Michaelides SA, Karachalios GN, et al. Pericardial involvement as an atypical manifestation of giant cell arteritis: report of a clinical case and literature review. Am J Med Sci 2006; 332:198.

[43] González-Gay MA, Ortego-Jurado M, Ercole L. et al. Giant cell arteritis: is the clinical spectrum of the disease changing? BMC Geriatr 2019; 200.

[44] Ritawa V, Temporal Arteritis. Ann Int Med 1951; 40: 63-87.

[45] Hernández-Rodríguez J, Tan CD, Molloy ES, et al. Vasculitis involving the breast: a clinical and histopathologic analysis of 34 patients. Medicine (Baltimore) 2008; 87:61.

Chapter 7

An Integrated Approach to the Role of Neurosonology in the Diagnosis of Giant Cell Arteritis

Dragoş Cătălin Jianu, Silviana Nina Jianu,
Georgiana Munteanu, Traian Flavius Dan,
Anca Elena Gogu and Ligia Petrica

Abstract

Giant cell arteritis (GCA) is a primary vasculitis that affects especially extra-cranial medium-sized arteries, such as superficial temporal arteries (TAs). Three findings are important for the ultrasound (US) diagnosis of TA: „dark halo" sign, which represents vessel wall edema, stenosis, and acute occlusions. US has a high sensitivity to detect vessel wall thickening in the case of large vessels GCA. The eye involvement in GCA is frequent and consists in arteritic anterior ischemic optic neuropathies or central retinal arterial occlusion, with abrupt, painless, and severe loss of vision of the involved eye. Because findings of TAs US do not correlate with eye complications in GCA, color Doppler imaging of the orbital vessels is of critical importance (it reveals low end diastolic velocities, and high resistance index), in order to quickly differentiate the mechanism of eye involvement (arteritic, versus non-arteritic). The former should be treated promptly with systemic corticosteroids to prevent further visual loss of the fellow eye.

Keywords: giant cell arteritis (GCA), temporal arteries (TAs), temporal artery biopsy (TAB), "dark halo" sign, ultrasonography (US), arteritic anterior ischemic optic neuropathies (A-AION), central retinal artery occlusion (CRAO), color Doppler imaging (CDI) of the orbital vessels, end diastolic velocities (EDV), resistance index (RI)

1. Introduction

Giant cell arteritis (GCA) is a primary (non-necrotizing granulomatous) vasculitis of autoimmune etiology, which especially affects extra cranial medium-sized arteries (branches of the external carotid arteries-ECAs-particularly the superficial temporal arteries-TAs) and sometimes large-sized arteries (aorta and its major branches). It is also recognized as Horton, temporal, or granulomatous arteritis. It causes narrowing of the artery, leading (by wall thickening) to partial (stenosis) or complete obstruction (occlusion) of local arterial blood flow, its clinical manifestations being expressed by signs of local ischemia [1–6].

GCA is the most common form of vasculitis that occurs in adults and in the elderly, being diagnosed over the age of 50's. Women are two to three times more affected than men. It is well known that the disease can occur in every racial group but is most common in Caucasians, especially people of northern European descent, and others in northern latitudes [1–6].

According to Hunder [7], and Jennette [8] a complete diagnosis of GCA requires the presence of American College of Rheumatology (ACR) classification modified criteria:

a. age over 50 years at the onset of the disease;

b. moderate, bitemporal, recently installed headache;

c. scalp tenderness, abnormal temporal arteries on inspection and palpation (**Figure 1**), reduced pulse, jaw claudication (pain in the jaw while/after chewing);

d. blurred vision or permanent visual loss in one or both eyes (since permanent visual loss due to ischemia is frequent, GCA should be considered an ophthalmic emergency requiring immediate management);

e. systemic symptoms (fatigue, weight loss, fever, pain in the shoulders and hips: polymyalgia rheumatica);

f. increased inflammatory markers (erythrocyte sedimentation rate greater than 50 mm/h, C reactive protein greater than 1,5 mg/dl);

g. representative histologic findings in temporal artery biopsy (TAB): mononuclear cell infiltration or granulomatous inflammation of the vessel wall, usually accompanied with multinucleated giant cells (**Figure 2**).

Several imaging techniques may be suitable in the diagnosis of GCA [9]. Compared to other imaging techniques, US is considered to be the most suitable in the evaluation of GCA patients, therefor it can easily be performed by the clinician (immediately after the general examination of patient), and it is significantly shortening the waiting period until another investigation is performed [9–16].

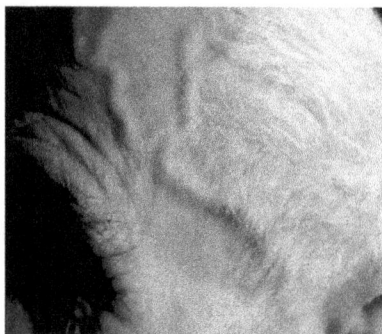

Figure 1.
Giant cell arteritis (GCA) of the left superficial temporal artery (TA) shows a prominent, tender and nodular artery, that is also hypo pulsating on palpation [9].

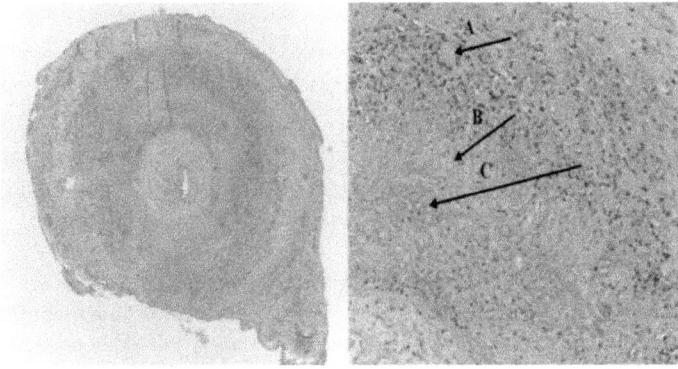

Figure 2.
The histopathological examination of the left superficial temporal artery biopsy (TAB) noted [10].
(A) Thickened vascular wall with inflammatory infiltration of multinucleated giant cells, (B) epithelioid cells
and (C) dissolution of the internal elastic lamina (H&E stain).

2. Extracranial duplex sonography in giant cell arteritis (GCA)

Ultrasonography (US) is a safe, noninvasive, without radiations, widespread accessible, fast, and low-cost bedside screening technique which has the unique capacity of studying real-time hemodynamics. It presents the ability to evaluate the anatomy of vessel's wall, identifying equally parietal abnormalities (wall thickening, hypoechoic plaques, clotting, parietal hematoma, dissections) and the external diameter of the artery; it can rule out both stenosis and occlusion. Therefore, the use of US is widespread in neurological clinical practice, mainly in the evaluation of arterial atherosclerotic process but also for monitoring other diseases such as medium/large-vessel vasculitis [17–19].

Olah noted that for US imaging of extracranial vessels different modes are being used:

a. *B-mode (brightness mode)*

- The strength of the echo is recorded as a bright dot, while the location of different gray dots corresponds to the depth of the target [17].

b. *The duplex image*

- It associates a B-mode gray-scale image with pulse-wave (PW) Doppler flow velocities measurements.

- The B-mode image represents the anatomical localization of the vessels, indicating the zone of interest where a Doppler sample volume should be placed and where the velocities are measured.

- The Doppler angle can be measured correctly when the blood is parallel to the direction of the vessel [17].

c. *Color Doppler flow imaging*

- Measure mean frequency shift in each sample volume.

- It represents color–coded velocity information, which is superimposed as a color flow map on a B-mode image.

- In each sample volume, the color reflects the blood flow velocity in a semi quantitative manner, as well as the flow direction relative to the transducer. Blood flowing toward or away from the transducer is shown by different colors (red and blue). Moreover, fast flow is indicated by a lighter hue and slow flow by a deeper one.

- The color flow map indicates the position and orientation of the vessels, as well as the site of turbulent flow or stenosis. Since color flow mapping is based on flow velocity measured by PW technology, aliasing occurs if the frequency shift is higher than half of the pulse repetition frequency (PRF) [17].

d.*Power Doppler mode*

- Uses the signal intensity of the returning Doppler signal instead of frequency shift.

- Power (intensity) of the signal is displayed as a color map superimposed on a B-mode image. Since the Doppler power is determined mainly by the volume rather than the velocity of moving blood, power Doppler imaging is free from aliasing artifacts and much more sensitive to detect flow, especially in the low-flow regions. However, it does not contain information about the flow direction or flow velocity [17].

The advantages of US over other imaging techniques in GCA are represented by its safety, accessibility, tolerability, fast (may take about 15-20 minutes, if it's conducted by an experienced sonographer) and the more important, its high resolution (a high –frequency probe offers both an axial and a lateral resolution of 0.1 mm) [19–27]. The smaller the vessel diameter, the more difficult is to appreciate the vessel wall damages, so that, in this case, the most informative US data are based on Doppler spectral evaluation. This is also valid for the assessment of medium to small vessel inflammation such as intracranial vasculitis. Small vessel vasculitis (the ANCA-associated or the immune complex vasculitis) are not a domain of ultrasound [19].

Furthermore, US has a higher sensitivity than TAB, the last one evaluating only a restricted anatomical region in a systemic disease. Using US, we can reveal pathological characteristics in GCA: non-compressible arteries (compression sign), the wall thickening ("halo" sign), stenosis and vessel occlusion. A normal intima-media complex (IMC) of an artery is represented by US as a homogeneous, hypoechoic or anechoic echo structure delineated by two parallel hyperechoic margins [19–27].

There is imperative to underline the importance of establishing the arteries that should be routinely examined in a patient suspected for GCA and these are: the TAs, and axillary arteries. If US of these arteries does not reveal suggestive lesions, in the presence of a clear patient history and of an obvious clinical examination, other arteries should be examined: other branches of the ECAs (the internal maxillary, the facial, the lingual, the occipital arteries), the vertebral, the subclavian, the common carotid arteries-CCAs, and the internal carotid arteries-ICAs [9, 19, 21].

Regarding the adequate US equipment for the diagnosis of GCA, modern high-resolution linear probes providing Doppler mode should be used, especially for examination of TAs. We should take into consideration that tissue penetration increases with lower frequencies and the resolution of US increases with higher frequencies. Probes that provide frequencies >20 MHz allow the clearly visualization of the normal IMC of TAs probes with frequencies ≥15 MHz are usually used for detection of minor wall thickening [19, 21].

2.1 Ultrasonography (US) of the large cervical and cervico-brachial vessels

In 2012, during the Chapel Hill Consensus Conference [19, 28], large vascular vasculitis (LVV) was well-defined as a vasculitis involving the aorta and its major branches, although any size of artery may be affected. This definition does not state that LVV mainly affects large vessels because in many patients, the number of medium and small arteries affected is greater than the number of large arteries involvement. For example, in GCA, only few branches of the ECAs may be affected when there is involvement of numerous small branches extending into the eye and orbit (e.g., central retinal artery, posterior ciliary arteries) [29, 30]. Less frequently, the CCA and the ICA are also affected (**Figures 3** and **4**) [9].

As Sturzenegger pointed up, angiography is not able to illustrate the vessel wall, so as to diagnose the inflammation of the large cervical and cervico-brachial vessels (aorta and its supra-aortic branches), the US can be very useful, since it can define alterations of the vessel wall with the use of B-mode imaging, while Doppler spectral flow velocity evaluation can help identify the stenosis or occlusion of the vessel [19].

Color Doppler Duplex sonography (CDDS) is an excellent device used in screening the large vessels involvement. Agreeing with different authors, including Sturzenegger, there are two ultra-sonographic hallmarks of large vessels GCA:

1. Vessel wall thickening, that typically is homogeneous, circumferential and over long segments (**Figures 4** and **5**);

2. Stenosis, typically revealing slickly tapered luminal tightening (hour glass like) [19–27]

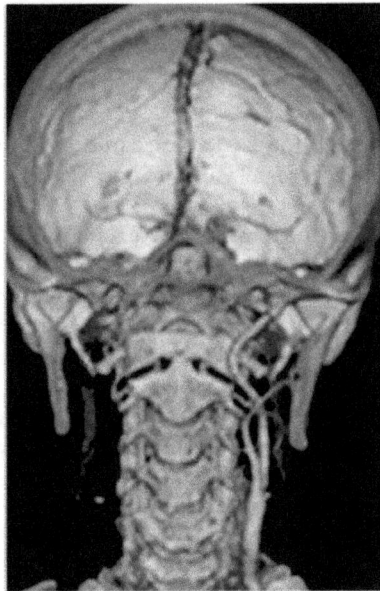

Figure 3.
Large vessels GCA; CT-angiography- occlusion of the left CCA, ECA, and ICA [9].

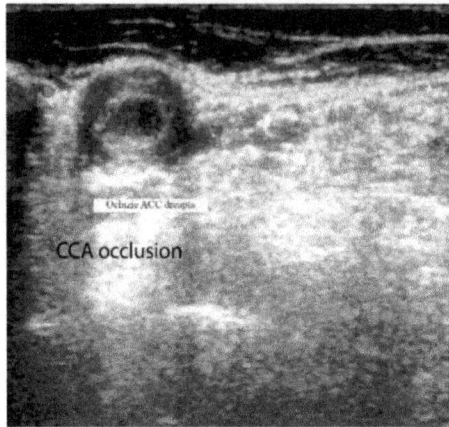

Figure 4.
Large vessels GCA, color Doppler ultrasound in transverse view of the right CCA. Hypoechoic wall swelling with right CCA occlusion [9].

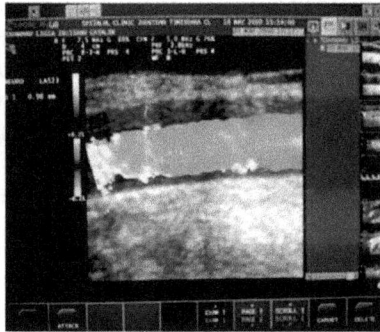

Figure 5.
Large vessel GCA, color Doppler ultrasound in longitudinal view of the right CCA with hypoechoic wall swelling [4].

Remarkably in some cases [9], the common carotid and the internal carotid arteries are also involved (large-vessel GCA) (**Figures 3–5**).

2.2 Ultrasonography (US) of the temporal arteries (TAs)

Extracranial Duplex sonography investigates almost completely the whole length of the common superficial TAs, including the frontal and parietal branches, and founds that inflammation is segmental (intermittent arterial involvement) [19–27]. The common superficial TA derives from the ECA. It divides into the frontal and parietal ramus in front of the ear. The distal common superficial TA and the rami are localized between the two layers of the temporal fascia, which is like a bright band at ultrasound examination [19–27].

2.2.1 Technical requirements

High-resolution color Doppler US can illustrate the vessel wall and the lumen of the TAs. One should use linear probes with a minimum gray scale frequency of 8 Mhz. Color frequency should be about 10 Mhz [19–27].

2.2.2 Machine adjustments

The pulse repetition frequency (PRF) should be about 2.5 kHz as maximum systolic velocities are rather high (20-100 cm/s). Steering of the color box and the Doppler beam should be maximal as the rami are parallel to the probe. It is important that the color covers the artery lumen exactly [19–27].

2.2.3 Sonographer training

The sonographer should perform at least 50 Duplex ultrasound of the TAs of subjects without GCA to be sure about the appearance of normal TAs before starting to evaluate patients with GCA [19–27].

2.2.4 Sequence of the ultrasound examination

The investigation should begin with the TA, using the longitudinal scan. The probe should then be moved along the course of the TA to the parietal ramus. On the way back one should delineate the TA in transverse scans. Using the transverse scan, one can find the frontal ramus, which should then be delineated in both scans (longitudinal and transverse). If the color signal indicates localized aliasing and diastolic flow, one should use the pw-Doppler mode to confirm the presence of stenosis [19–27].

In 1997 Schmidt et al. proved that the most specific (almost 100% specificity) and sensitive (73% sensitivity) sign for GCA was a concentric hypo-echogenic mural thickening, dubbed "halo", which the authors interpreted as "vessel wall edema" [24].

Other positive findings for GCA are the presence of occlusion and stenosis [19–27].

In conclusion, there are three important items in the ultrasound diagnosis of temporal arteritis:

a. "dark halo" sign – a typically homogeneous, hypoechoic, circumferential wall thickening around the lumen of an inflamed TA - which represents vessel wall edema and a characteristic finding in temporal arteritis/GCA. It is well delineated toward the lumen (**Figure 6**).

b. stenosis are documented by blood-flow velocities, which are more than twice the rate recorded in the area of stenosis compared with the area before the stenosis, with wave forms demonstrating turbulence and reduced velocities behind the area of stenosis (**Figure 7**).

c. acute occlusions, in which the US image is comparable to that of acute embolism in other vessels, showing hypoechoic material in the former artery lumen with absence of color signals [19–27].

Related ultrasound patterns can be found in other arteries: the facial, the internal maxillary, the lingual, the occipital, the distal subclavian and the axillary arteries.

The best time to perform ultrasound investigation is before initiating the corticosteroid treatment, or in the first 7 days of treatment, since with corticosteroid therapy the" halo" revealed by TAs ultrasound disappears within 2-3 weeks. The wall inflammation, stenosis, or occlusions of the larger arteries (CCA, ICA) remain for months, despite corticosteroid treatment. However, the diagnosis process should not postpone the initiation of therapy. Ultrasound may also detect inflamed

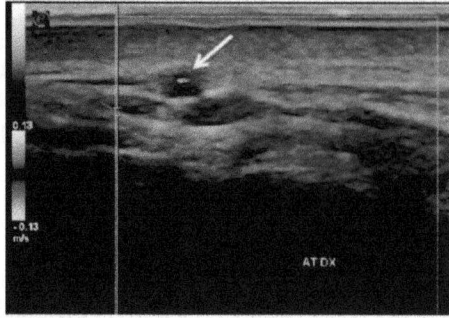

Figure 6.
Color Doppler ultrasonography (CDUS) of the right TA shows a hypoechoic halo around the lumen in transverse view (arrow). The "halo sign" corresponds to edema of the artery wall [11].

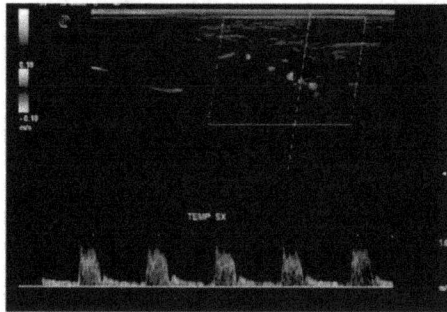

Figure 7.
Longitudinal view of the right TA by color Doppler ultrasonography (CDUS) shows a hypoechoic halo of the TA and the presence of turbulent and weak flow, suggesting the presence of stenosis. The PSV is 1 m/s, that is double compared to the segment without stenosis [11].

TAs in patients with clinically normal TAs. Some patients with the clinical image of polymyalgia rheumatica, but with hidden TAs may be diagnosed using ultrasonography [9–16, 19–27].

In 2010, Arida et al. [26] evaluated a number of studies that examined the sensitivity and specificity of the "halo" sign confirmed by TA ultrasound (US) for GCA diagnosis versus the American College of Rheumatology (ACR) 1990 criteria for the classification of this vasculitis (used as a reference standard). Only 8 studies involving 575 patients, 204 of whom received the final diagnosis of GCA, achieved the technical quality criteria for US. This meta-analysis disclosed a sensitivity of 68% and a specificity of 91% for the unilateral "halo" sign, as well as 43% and 100%, respectively, for the bilateral "halo" sign in TA US for GCA diagnosis when the 1990 ACR criteria are used as the reference standard. The authors established that the halo sign in US is of great utility in diagnosing GCA [19–27].

In the case of consistent clinical and sonographic results, temporal arteries biopsy (TAB) does not appear to be useful and justified [19, 27].

Sturzenegger affirmed that differential diagnosis with arteriosclerosis is important in patients over 50 years, taking into consideration that GCA with large vessels disease disturbs almost exclusively this category of patients. There are some characteristic features of the arteriosclerotic wall: the thickening usually appears less homogeneous; there are calcified arteriosclerotic plaques ulcers; stenosis extends over shorter segments, they are not concentric, not tapering, and location of lesions differs (e.g., mainly bifurcations) [19].

Besides, agreeing to Sturzenegger, differential diagnosis with the other LVV, especially Takayasu arteritis, has to be reflected:

- Takayasu arteritis usually affects women below the age of 40 years;

- symptoms like tender scalp or polymyalgia syndrome are exceptional;

- the involvement of CCA is more frequent in Takayasu arteritis, while the involvement of temporal artery in Takayasu arteritis is not known;

- US image of wall thickening ("halo") is brighter in TA than in GCA probably due to a larger mural edema in GCA which is a more acute disease than TA. Reflected [19–27].

2.3 Color Doppler imaging (CDI) of orbital (retro-bulbar) vessels

Approximately 25% of patients with temporal artery biopsy (TAB) - proven GCA have ophthalmologic complications: usually unilateral visual loss (due to the vasculitic involvement of orbital vessels:

a. of posterior ciliary arteries (PCAs) - represented by arteritic anterior ischemic optic neuropathies (A-AION), or

b. of central retinal artery (CRA) - represented by central retinal artery occlusion (CRAO) [31–35].

Schmidt compared the results of TAs-US examinations with the occurrence of visual ischemic complications (A-AION, CRAO, branch retinal artery occlusion, diplopia, or amaurosis fugax) in 222 consecutive patients with newly diagnosed, active GCA [21–24].
However, findings of TAs US did not correlate with eye complications [21–24].
This is the reason why we always have to exam the orbital (retrobulbar) vessels in GCA patients or in patients with unilateral abrupt visual loss [9–16] (**Figure 8A,B**).

2.3.1 Orbital (retrobulbar) vessels

The ophthalmic artery (OA) branches in several arteries, including (**Table 1**):

a. the central retinal artery (CRA) (**Figure 8 A**), and

b. the posterior ciliary arteries (nasal and temporal branches-nPCAs, tPCAs) [28, 31, 32] (**Figure 8B**), (**Table 1**) [15, 28, 31, 32].

OA finishes in the a. supra-trohlearis and *A. dorsalis* nasi.

2.3.2 Probe selection

Standard neurovascular ultrasound machines equipped with linear-array transducers emitting 6-12 MHz (up to 15 MHz) are adequate for identifying (by Color Doppler sonography), and measuring (by spectral analysis pulsed Doppler sonography) the blood flow in the orbital vessels: the OA, the CRA and central retinal vein (CRV), PCAs, and the superior ophthalmic vein (SOV) [28, 31, 32].

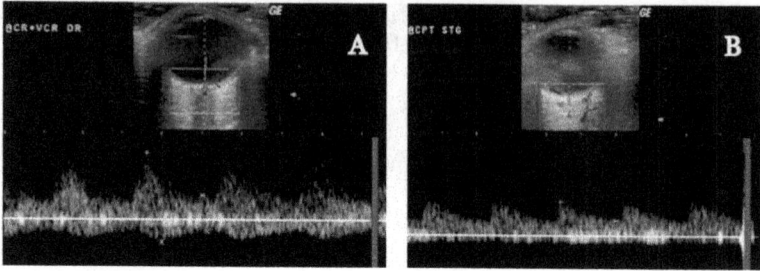

Figure 8.
Color Doppler imaging (CDI) of orbital (retro-bulbar) vessels: (A). central retinal artery (CRA); (B). posterior ciliary arteries (PCAs) [15].

Parameter	OA	CRA	PCA (temporal)	PCA (nasal)	SOV (superior ophthalmic vein)
PSV (cm/s)	45,3 ± 10,5	17,3 ± 2,6	13,3 ± 3,5	12,4 ± 3,4	10,2 ± 3,8
EDV (cm/s)	11,8 ± 4,3	6,2 ± 2,7	6,4 ± 1,5	5,8 ± 2,5	4,3 ± 2,4
RI	0,74 ± 0,07	0,63 ± 0,09	0,52 ± 0,10	0,53 ± 0,08	

Note: These are the normal flow velocities and resistances index in orbital vessels which are generally accepted by the specialists.

Table 1.
Normal flow velocities and Resistance Index in orbital vessels [15, 31, 32].

The CRA, a distal branch of the OA, enters the optic nerve (ON) approximately 1-1.5 cm distal from the bulbus coming from the dorsolateral direction. Parallel to this is the CRV.

The PCAs are located near the optic nerve (ON) (the nasal-nPCA and the temporal-tPCA branches) [28, 31, 32].

If the vessels are difficult to display, the power should be elevated for a short time if the clinical question is important [28, 31, 32].

2.3.3 Arterial blood supply of the anterior part of the optic nerve

The optic nerve head (ONH) consists of (from anterior to posterior):

a. the surface nerve fiber layer - mostly supplied by the retinal arterioles. The cilioretinal artery, when present, usually supplies the corresponding sector of the surface layer [36–40].

b. the prelaminar region - situated anterior of the lamina cribrosa. It is supplied by centripetal branches from the peripapillary choroid [36–40].

c. the lamina cribrosa region - supplied by centripetal branches from the posterior ciliary arteries (PCAs), either directly or by the so-called arterial circle of Zinn and Haller (when is present) [36–40].

d. the retrolaminar region - is the part of the ONH that lies immediately behind the lamina cribrosa. It is supplied by two vascular systems: the peripheral centripetal and the axial centrifugal systems. The previous represents the main source of stream for this part. It is formed by recurrent pial branches arising from the peripapillary choroid and the circle of Zinn and Haller (when present, or the PCAs instead). In addition, pial branches from the central retinal artery (CRA) also supply this part. The latter is not present in all eyes. When present, it is formed by inconstant branches arising from the intraneural part of the CRA.

From the description of the arterial supply of the ONH given above, it is obvious that the PCAs are the main source of blood supply to the ONH [36–40].

2.3.4 Pathophysiology of factors controlling blood flow in the optic nerve head (ONH)

The blood flow in the ONH depends upon [36–40]:

a. resistance to blood flow - depends upon the condition and caliber of the vessels supplying the ONH, which in turn are influenced by: the efficiency of auto-regulation of the ONH blood flow, the vascular variations in the arteries feeding the ONH circulation, and the rheological properties of the blood.

b. arterial blood pressure (BP) - both arterial hypertension and hypotension can influence the ONH blood flow in several ways. In an ONH, a fall of blood pressure below a critical level of auto-regulation would decrease its blood flow. Decrease of BP in the ONH may be due to systemic (nocturnal arterial hypotension during sleep, intensive antihypertensive medication, etc.) or local hypotension.

c. intra-ocular pressure (IOP) - there is an opposite relationship between intra-ocular pressure and perfusion pressure in the ONH.

The blood flow in the ONH is calculated by using the following formula:

Perfusion pressure = Mean BP minus intraocular pressure (IOP).
Mean BP = Diastolic BP + 1/3 (systolic - diastolic BP) [6, 13].

3. Anterior ischemic optic neuropathies (AIONs)

AION is the consequence of an acute ischemic disorder (a segmental infarction) of the ONH supplied by the PCAs. Blood supply interruption can occur with or without arterial inflammation. Therefore, AION is of two types: non-arteritic AION (NA-AION) and arteritic AION (A-AION). The prior is far more common than the last, and they are distinct entities etiologically, pathogenically, clinically and from the management point of view [36–40].

A history of amaurosis fugax before an abrupt, painless, and severe loss of vision of the involved eye, with concomitant diffuse pale optic disc edema is extremely suggestive of A-AION. None of these symptoms are found in NA-AION patients [36–40].

3.1 Spectral Doppler analysis of the orbital (retro-bulbar) vessels in A-AION

In acute stage, blood flow cannot be detected in the PCAs in the clinically affected eye of any of the GCA patients with A-AION. Low end diastolic velocities (EDV) and high resistance index (RI) are identified in all other orbital vessels (including the PCAs in the opposite eye) of all A-AION patients [9–14, 41].

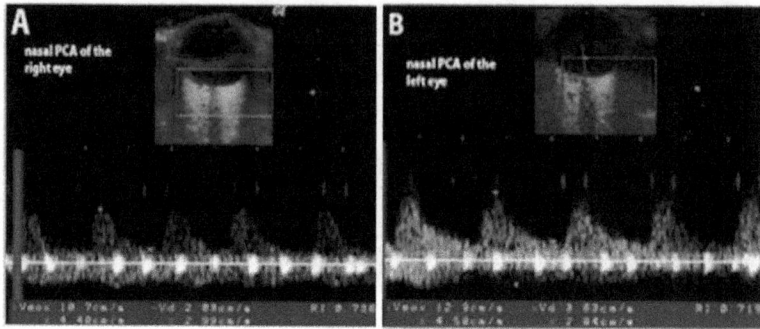

Figure 9.
CDI of the PCAs in A-AION: (A). Decreased EDV in the nasal PCAs of the clinically affected right eye, and (B) of the clinically unaffected left eye.

Over 7 days, Spectral Doppler analysis of the orbital vessels highlights blood flow alterations in all A-AION patients even with a high-dose corticosteroids therapy. Severely reduced blood flow velocities (especially EDV) in the PCAs of the affected eye (both nasal and temporal branches), compared to the unaffected eye, are observed. An increased RI in the PCAs is noted (the RI is higher on the clinically affected eye as compared to the unaffected eye) [9–14, 41] (**Figure 9A,B**).

Fewer abnormalities are detected in the CRAs: high RI are measured in both sides, with decreased peak systolic velocities (PSV) in the CRA of the clinically affected eye [9–14, 41].

Similar abnormalities are noted in the OAs: high RI are measured in both sides [9–14, 41].

At 1 month, after treatment with high-dose corticosteroids, CDI examinations of orbital blood vessels reveals that blood flow normalization is slow in all A-AION patients [9–14, 41].

In conclusion, the Spectral Doppler Analysis of the orbital vessels in A-AION indicates (after several days of corticosteroid treatment) low blood velocities, especially EDV, and high RI in all orbital vessels, in both orbits. These signs represent characteristic signs of the CDI of the orbital vessels in A-AION [9–14, 41].

3.2 Spectral Doppler analysis of the orbital (retro-bulbar) vessels in NA-AION

In contrast, the patients with NA-AION present the following characteristics in acute stage, and at 1 week of evolution:

- minor reduction of PSV in PCAs (nasal and temporal) in the affected eye, compared to the unaffected eye.

- slight decrease of PSV in CRA of the affected eye, due to papillary edema [9–14, 41]:

- in OAs, PSV are variable: normal to decreased, according to ipsilateral ICAs status.

Severe ICA stenosis (≥70% of vessel diameter) combined with an insufficient Willis polygon led to diminish PSV in ipsilateral OA [9–14, 41].

In 1 month, CDI examinations of orbital blood vessels reveal that blood flow normalization is reached. The exceptions are the cases with severe ipsilateral ICA stenosis/occlusion [9–14, 41].

In conclusion, in NA-AION, blood velocities and RI in PCAs are preserved. Similar results were obtained in other studies [9–14, 41].

Fluorescein angiogram and CDI of the orbital vessels data support the histo-pathological evidence of involvement of the entire trunk of the PCAs in the A-AION (impaired optic disc and choroidal perfusion in the patients with A-AION). On the other hand, in the NA-AION, the impaired flow to the optic nerve head (ONH) is distal to the PCAs themselves, possibly at the level of the para-optic branches (only 1/3 of the flow of the PCAs) [36–40].

These branches supply the ONH directly (impaired optic disc perfusion, with relatively conservation of the choroidal perfusion) [36–40].

Extremely delayed or absent filling of the choroid has been depicted as a fluo-rescein angiogram characteristic of arteritic AION and has been suggested as one useful factor by which A-AION can be differentiated from NA-AION [36–40].

4. Central retinal artery occlusion (CRAO)

CRAO is the result of an abrupt diminuation of blood flow in CRA, severe enough to cause ischemia of the inner retina. Due to the fact that there are no functional anastomoses between choroidal (PCAs) and retinal circulation (CRA), CRAO determines severe and permanent loss of vision. Therefore, it is very important to identify the cause of CRAO, in order to protect the contralateral eye. Frequently, the site of the blockage is within the optic nerve substance and for this reason, it is generally not visible on the ophthalmoscopy. The majority of CRAO are caused by thrombus formation due to systemic diseases, including GCA. For this reason, all patients with CRAO should undergo a systemic evaluation [42–44].

4.1 Spectral Doppler analysis of the orbital (retro-bulbar) vessels in CRAO

The patients with an unilateral CRAO present at the Spectral Doppler analysis of the retrobulbar vessels the following aspects [9, 15, 16]:

a. an elevated RI in the CRAs (the RI is higher on the affected side, than it is on the unaffected side); with severe diminished blood flow velocities (especially EDV) in the CRA.

b. fewer abnormalities are observed in the PCAs, and in the OAs (**Figure 10**).

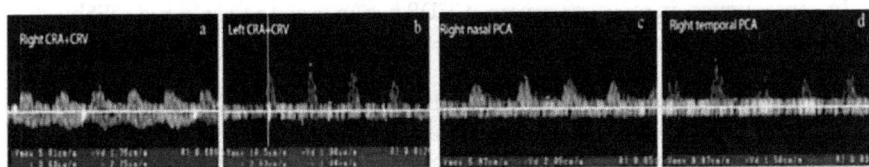

Figure 10.
CDI of orbital vessels revealed severely diminished EDV and high RI in both CRAs (a, b) despite the fact that the left eye had the normal aspect at ophthalmoscopy. Fewer abnormalities were observed in the PCAs (c, d) [15].

5. US and others imaging techniques

Other imaging techniques, such as high-resolution magnetic resonance imaging (MRI), magnetic resonance-angiography (MR-A), computer tomography angiography (CT-A), positron emission tomography (PET) provide valuable information regarding the structure of large vessels, highlighting with much greater precision the thoracic aorta, compared with US [45–47].

There are few studies that compared US with other imaging techniques. Some of them indicated that there is a good correlation between US and PET, even though PET might have a little more sensitivity for vertebral arteries examination [45–46]. 18F-fluorodeoxyglucose-positron emission tomography/ computed tomography (FDG-PET/CT) has a higher sensitivity for detection of large arteries and aortic involvement - analysis of the arterial wall [45, 46]. The diagnostic power of high-resolution MRI and color-coded duplex US of extra-cranial arteries in detecting GCA are equivalent [47].

The disadvantages of this techniques are: they are more expensive, hardly accessible, some of them are limited by invasiveness, nephrotoxicity (angiography) and exposure to high radiations (CT,PET), this is why they might be unnecessary (excepting those patients with exclusively thoracic aorta involvement) and are not accepted as diagnostic methods in GCA. They should only be used when interventions are required [45–47].

All these imaging techniques should always be performed by well-trained specialists, using suitable equipment and operational protocols [45–47].

Nevertheless, US is particularly useful in examining the orbital vessels [9–16, 28, 31, 32, 41].

The diagnostic work-up of AION benefits from the combined used of fluorescein angiography and noninvasive multimodal imaging, including CDI of the orbital vessels and structural Optical Coherence Tomography (OCT) of the optic nerve head (ONH) and OCT angiography [10, 48]. They provide very detailed information regarding the structural (retinal nerve fiber layer-RNFL-thickness/optic disc edema) and vascular impairments (microvascular defects-vessel tortuosity, and vessel density reduction) of the ONH, respectively [10, 48].

6. Conclusions

US should be used as a first-line diagnostic investigation for patients presenting with clinical and biological features suggestive for GCA, taking into consideration that it has a high sensitivity to detect vessel wall thickening (dark hallo sign) in the case of large/medium vessels. In a few cases of our studies, the CCAs and the ICAs were also involved.

In consequence, in our department, CCDS has emerged as a safe and reliable alternative to TAB as a point of care diagnostic tool in the management of temporal arteritis.

The eye involvement in GCA is frequent and consists in A-AIONs or CRAO, with abrupt, painless, and severe loss of vision of the involved eye.

Because findings of TAs US do not correlate with eye complications in GCA, CDI of the orbital vessels is of critical importance, in order to quickly differentiate the mechanism of eye involvement (arteritic, versus non-arteritic). This US tehnique may be helpful to detect the blood flow in the orbital vessels, especially in cases of opacity of the medium, or when the clinical appearance of ophthalmologic complications in temporal arteritis is athypical.

The Spectral Doppler Analysis of the orbital vessels in GCA with eye involvement reveals low blood velocities, especially EDV, and high RI in all orbital vessels, in both orbits, for all patients (especially on the affected side).

A huge advantage of CDI of orbital vessels is that it provides immediate information that can be used to inform treatment decisions, including a potential reduction in loss of sight and avoidance of unnecessary long-term steroid treatment by early exclusion of mimics.

Author details

Dragoş Cătălin Jianu[1,2*], Silviana Nina Jianu[3], Georgiana Munteanu[2],
Traian Flavius Dan[1,2], Anca Elena Gogu[1,2] and Ligia Petrica[4]

1 Department of Neurology, "Victor Babes" University of Medicine and Pharmacy, Timisoara, Romania

2 Department of Neurology, Clinical Emergency County Hospital, Timisoara, Romania

3 Department of Ophthalmology, Military Emergency Hospital, Timisoara, Romania

4 Department of Nephrology, "Victor Babes" University of Medicine and Pharmacy, Timisoara, Romania

*Address all correspondence to: dcjianu@yahoo.com

IntechOpen

References

[1] Gonzalez-Gay M.(2005) The diagnosis and management of patients with giant cell arteritis. *J Rheumatol* 2005;32:1186-1188.

[2] Salvarani C, Cantini F, Hunder GG (2008): Polymyalgia rheumatica and giant-cell arteritis. *Lancet* 2008, 372:234-245.

[3] Melson MR, Weyand CM, Newman NJ, Biousse V. The diagnosis of giant cell arteritis. Rev Neurol Dis 2007: 4(3): 128 - 42.

[4] Hayreh SS, Podhajsky PA, Raman R, Zimmerman B. Giant cell arteritis: validity and reliability of various diagnostic criteria. AmJOphthalmol 1997: 123(3): 285- 96.

[5] Levine SM, Hellmann DB. (2002) Giant cell arteritis. Curr Opin Rheumatol 2002;14:3-10.

[6] Gonzalez-Gay MA, Vazquez-Rodriguez TR, Lopez-Diaz MJ, et al. Epidemiology of giant cell arteritis and polymyalgia rheumatica Arthritis Rheum 2009, 61:1454-1461.

[7] Hunder G.G., et al. (1990) - The American College of Reumatology 1990 criteria for the classification of giant cell arteritis, Arteritis Rheum. 1990; 33:1122-28.

[8] Jennette J et al-Revised international Chapell Hill consensus Conference Nomenclature of Vasculitides. Arthritis Rheum. 2013;65:1-11.

[9] Jianu DC, Jianu SN, Petrica L, Serpe M - Advances in the Diagnosis and Treatment of Vasculitis - Luis M Amezcua-Guerra (Ed.)-Chapter 16, Large Giant Cell Arteritis with Eye Involvement, InTech, Rijeka, Croatia,2011, pg 311-330.

[10] Stanca HT, Suvac E, Munteanu M, Jianu DC, Motoc AGM, Rosca GC,

Boruga O - Giant cell arteritis with arteritic anterior ischemic optic neuropathy. Rom J Morphol Embryol 2017, 58 (1): 281-285.

[11] Jianu DC, Jianu SN. Chapter 8-The role of Color Doppler Imaging in the study of optic neuropathies. In: Jianu DC, Jianu SN, editors. Color Doppler Imaging. Neuro-ophthalmological correlations. Timisoara, Romania: Mirton: 2010. p. 154- 74.

[12] Jianu DC, Jianu SN– Updates in the diagnosis and treatment of vasculitis - Lazaros Sakkas and Christina Katsiari (Ed.) - Chapter 5, Giant Cell Arteritis and arteritic anterior ischemic optic neuropathies InTech, Rijeka, Croatia, 2013, pg 111- 130.

[13] Jianu DC, Jianu SN, Petrica L, Motoc AGM, Dan TF, Lazureanu DC, Munteanu M - Clinical and color Doppler imaging features of one patient with occult giant cell arteritis presenting arteritic anterior ischemic optic neuropathy. Rom J Morphol Embryol 2016, 57(2): 579-583.

[14] Jianu DC, Jianu SN, Munteanu M, Petrica L-Clinical and ultrasonographic features in anterior ischemic optic neuropathies –Vojnosanitetski Pregled (Military Medical and Pharmaceutical Journal of Serbia) 2018, August, Vol.75 (No.8): p.773-779.

[15] Jianu DC, Jianu SN. Chapter 6-The role of Color Doppler Imaging in the study of central retinal artery obstruction. In: Jianu DC, Jianu SN, editors. Color Doppler Imaging. Neuro-ophthalmological correlations. Timisoara, Romania: Mirton: 2010. p. 125-142.

[16] Jianu DC, Jianu SN, Munteanu M, Vlad D, Rosca C, Petrica L - Color Doppler imaging features of two patients presenting central retinal artery occlusion with and without giant

cell arteritis. Vojnosanitetski Pregled (Military Medical and Pharmaceutical Journal of Serbia) 2016 April Vol.73 (No.4), 397-401.

[17] Laszlo Olah. Chapter 1 Ultrasound principles pg 1-14, in Manual of Neurosonology, L Csiba, and C Baracchini (ed), Cambridge University Press, Cambridge, United Kingdom, 2016.

[18] Massimo Del Sete and Valentina Saia. Chapter 5A. Atherosclerotic carotid disease. Carotid ultrasound imaging, pg 57-63, in Manual of Neurosonology, L Csiba, and C Baracchini (ed), Cambridge University Press, Cambridge, United Kingdom, 2016.

[19] Mathias H. Sturzenegger. Chapter 8 Cervical artery vasculitides pg 300-305, in Manual of Neurosonology, L Csiba, and C Baracchini (ed), Cambridge University Press, Cambridge, United Kingdom, 2016).

[20] Duftner C, Dejaco C, Moller-Dohn U. Ultrasound definitions for vasculitis in cranial and large vessel giant cell arteritis: results of a Delphi survey of the OMERACT ultrasound large vessel vasculitis group. Ann Rheum Dis2016;75(Suppl 2):626. Doi:10.1136/annrheumdis-2016-eular.5487.

[21] Schmidt WA. Role of ultrasound in the understanding and management of vasculitis. Ther Adv Musculoskelet Dis 2014; 6: 39-47.

[22] Wolfgang A. Schmidt Ultrasound in the diagnosis and management of giant cell arteritis. Rheumatology 2018; 57: ii22-ii31 doi:10.1093/rheumatology/kex461.

[23] Schmidt WA.Takayasu and temporal arteritis, in Baumgartner R.W. (ed.): Handbook on Neurovascular Ultrasound. Front.Neurol.Neurosci. Basel, Karger, 2006, 21:96-104.

[24] Schmidt WA, Kraft HE, Vorpahl K, et al.Color duplex ultrasonography in the diagnosis of temporal arteritis. N Engl J Med 1997, 337:1336-1342.

[25] Monti S, Floris A, Ponte C et al. The use of ultrasound to assess giant cell arteritis: review of the current evidence and practical guide for the rheumatologist. Rheumatology 2018;57:227-35.

[26] Arida A, Kyprianou M, Kanakis M, Sfikakis PP. The diagnostic value of ultrasonography-derived edema of the temporal artery wall in giant cell arteritis: a second meta-analysis. BMC Musculoskelet Disord 2010, 11:44.

[27] Jared Ching, Sonja Mansfield Smith, Bhaskar Dasgupta, Erika Marie Damato, The Role of Vascular Ultrasound in Managing Giant Cell Arteritis in Ophthalmology https://doi.org/10.1016/j.survophthal.2019.11.004Get rights and content.

[28] Mario Siebler. Chapter 25 Neuro-orbital ultrasound, pg 300-305 in Manual of Neurosonology, L Csiba, and C Baracchini (ed), Cambridge University Press, Cambridge, United Kingdom, 2016).

[29] Martínez-Valle F, Solans-Laqué R, Bosch-Gil J, et al.(2010): Aortic involvement in giant cell arteritis. Autoimmun Rev 2010, 9:521-524.

[30] Agard C, Barrier JH, Dupas B, et al. Aortic involvement in recent-onset giant cell (temporal) arteritis: a case-control prospective study using helical aortic computed tomodensitometric scan. Arthritis Rheum 2008, 59:670-676.

[31] Pichot O, Gonzalvez B, Franco A, Mouillon M. Color Doppler ultrasonography in the study of orbital and ocular vascular diseases. J Fr Ophtalmol; 2001, 19(1): 19-31.

[32] Lieb WE, Cohen SM, Merton DA, Shields JA, Mitchell DG, Goldberg BB. Color Doppler imaging of the eye and orbit. Technique and normal vascular anatomy. Arch Ophthalmol 1991; 109(4): 527- 31.

[33] Gonzalez-Gay MA, Garcia-Porrua C, Llorca J, Hajeer AH, Branas F, Dababneh A, et al.(2000) Visual manifestations of giant cell arteritis: trends and clinical spectrum in 161 patients. Medicine (Baltimore) 2000;79:283-92.

[34] Singh AG, Kermani TA, Crowson CS, Weyand CM, Matteson EL, Warrington KJ. Visual manifestations in giant cell arteritis: Trend over 5 decades in a population-based cohort. J Rheumatol 2015: 42(2): 309-15.

[35] Hayreh SS, Podhajsky PA, Zimmerman B. Occult giant cell arteritis: ocular manifestations. Am J Ophthalmol 1998: 125(4): 521- 6.

[36] Biousse V: Newman NJ. Ischemic Optic Neuropathies. N Engl J Med 2015: 372(25): 2428- 36.

[37] Arnold AC.Chapter 191 - Ischemic optic neuropathy, in Ianoff M., Duker J.S., ed., Ophtalmology, second edition, Mosby, 2004:1268-1272.

[38] Collignon-Robe NJ, Feke GT, Rizzo JF. Optic nerve head circulation in nonarteritic anterior ischemic optic neuropathy and optic neuritis, Ophthalmol. 2004; 111: 1663-72.

[39] Hayreh SS. Ischemic optic neuropathies-where are we now? Graefes Arch Clin Exp Oplnhalmol 2013: 251(8): 1873-84.

[40] Hayreh SS. Management of ischemic optic neuropathies. Inidian J Ophthalmol 2011:59(2): 123- 36.

[41] Tranquart F, Aubert-Urena AS, Arsene S, Audrierie C, Rossazza C., Pourcelot L. Echo-Doppler couleur des arteres ciliaires posterieures dans la neuropathie optique ischemique anterieure aigue, J.E.MU. 1997; 18(1):6871.

[42] Duker JS. Chapter 114 - Retinal arterial obstruction, in Yanoff M., Duker J.S., ed., Ophtalmology, second edition, Mosby, 2004:856-63.

[43] Ahuja RM, Chaturvedi S, Elliot A, et al. Mechanism of retinal arterial occlusive disease in African, American and Caucasian patients, Stroke 1999, 30(8): 479-84.

[44] Connolly BP, Krishnan A, Shah GK, Whelan J, Brown GC, Eagle RC, et al. Characteristics of patients presenting with central retinal artery occlusion with and without giant cell arteritis. Can J Ophthalmol 2000; 35(7): 379-84.

[45] Czihal M, Tato F, Forster S et al. Fever of unknown origin as initial manifestation of large vessel giant cell arteritis: diagnosis by colour-coded sonography and 18-FDG-PET. Clin Exp Rheumatol 2010;28:549-52.

[46] Germano G, Macchioni P, Possemato N et al. Contrast enhanced ultrasound of the carotid artery in patients with large vessel vasculitis: correlation with positron emission tomography findings. Arthritis Care Res 2017;69:143-9.

[47] Bley TA, Reinhard M, Hauenstein C et al. Comparison of duplex sonography and high-resolution magnetic resonance imaging in the diagnosis of giant cell (temporal) arteritis. Arthritis Rheum 2008; 58: 2574-8.

[48] Pierro L, Arrigo A, Aragona E, Cavalleri M, Bandello F. Vessel Density and vessel tortuosity quantitative analysis of A-AIONS and NA-AIONS: an OCT-Angiography Study. Journal of Clinical Medicine 2020;Apr 12;9 (4)1094 doi: 10.3390/jcm9041094

www.ingramcontent.com/pod-product-compliance
Lightning Source LLC
Chambersburg PA
CBHW070241230326
41458CB00100B/5725